Priya Ilangovan.

May 92

ACUTE DIARRHEA

Its Nutritional Consequences in Children

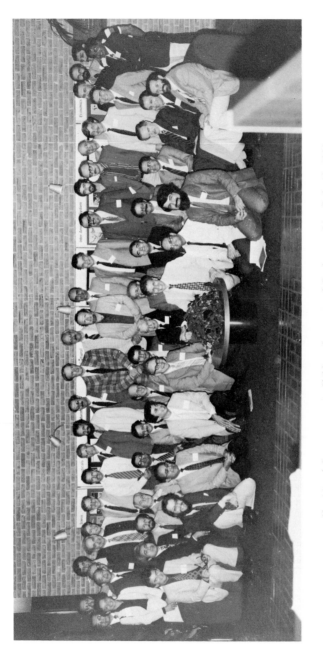

Nutritional Consequences in Children, International Conference, May 7, 8, 10, 1983

Back row: Liu Wen-Jang, Hilda Mejiias de Contreras, Raul Leon Barua, Huang, Father Josef Kadlec, Kenneth H. Brown, Albert Kapikian, Graeme Barnes, Richard Wyatt, Leonardo Mata, Robert Edelman, Gerald T. Keusch, Frederick T. Koster, Nathaniel Pierce, William J. Klish, R. Bradley Sack, Franklin de los Santos, Emanuel Lebenthal, David R. Nalin, Paul Offit, Karl Western, Robert H. Parrott, Robert E. Black, Oscar Brunser, John B. Robbins, Michael Salgo, José Cruz, M. Santosham. *Middle row:* H. Hilpert, Tasuke Konno, Guillermo Ruiz-Palacios, Edward Demaeyer, R. K. Chandra, Robert H. Yolken, Lars A. Hanson, Pearay L. Ogra, Mitchel I. Rubin, Benjamin José Schmidt, Pierre R. Guesry, Aderbal Sabra, José O. Mora, Rodrigo Crespo, Humberto Soriano, Myron Levine. *Front row:* Jorge Flores, R. V. Chaudhari, Rodrigo C. Hurtado, Robert M. Suskind, Joseph A. Bellanti, Angel R. Colon, Claudio Lanata.

Acute Diarrhea

Its Nutritional Consequences in Children

Editor

Joseph A. Bellanti, M.D.

*Professor of Pediatrics and Microbiology
Director, International Center for
Interdisciplinary Studies of Immunology
Georgetown University School of Medicine
Washington, D.C.*

Nestlé Nutrition
Workshop Series
Volume 2

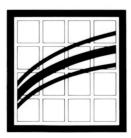

RAVEN PRESS ■ NEW YORK

Raven Press, 1140 Avenue of the Americas, New York, New York 10036

The material contained in this volume was submitted as previously unpublished material, except in the instances in which credit has been given to the source from which some of the illustrative material was derived.

Great care has been taken to maintain the accuracy of the information contained in the volume. However, Nestlé Nutrition and Raven Press cannot be held responsible for errors or for any consequences arising from the use of the information contained herein.

Materials appearing in this book prepared by individuals as part of their official duties as U.S. Government employees are not covered by the above-mentioned copyright.

Library of Congress Cataloging in Publication Data
Main entry under title:

Acute diarrhea.

Summary of an international workshop, sponsored by the
International Center for Interdisciplinary Studies of
Immunology at Georgetown University, Washington, D.C., on
May 7–10, 1982.
  Includes bibliographies and index.
  1. Diarrhea in children—Congresses.
2. Malnutrition in children—Congresses. I. Bellanti,
Joseph A., 1934–   . II. Georgetown University.
International Center for Interdisciplinary Studies of
Immunology. [DNLM: 1. Diarrhea, Infantile—Complications.
2. Nutrition disorders—In infancy and childhood.
WS 312 A189]
RJ456.D5A27   1983   618.92′3427   83-3290
ISBN 0-89004-991-2 (Raven Press)

Second Printing, June 1985

Preface

This volume is a summary of an international workshop, "Acute Diarrhea: Its Nutritional Consequences in Children," which was held in Washington, D.C., on May 7–10, 1982. The objective of the conference was to review the most recent advances in acute diarrhea in infancy, including aspects of epidemiology, pathogenesis, therapy, and prevention, and to emphasize the interactions between acute diarrhea and malnutrition in both the industrialized and the developing countries of the world. Over 50 internationally recognized researchers contributed to the workshop from such diverse countries as Japan, Honduras, Brazil, Switzerland, Czechoslovakia, Peru, Costa Rica, Germany, Colombia, Venezuela, Mexico, Uruguay, Chile, Canada, and the United States.

The volume opens with a broad overview of the epidemiology of acute diarrhea in childhood and summarizes the experiences of a large number of field studies that have examined public health, epidemiologic, socioeconomic, and cultural factors contributing to the transmission of disease-producing pathogens. The volume progresses to a discussion of the etiologic agents of acute diarrhea including the newer viral, bacterial, and parasitic agents. Of particular interest in this regard is the new information concerning the recognition of various strains of rotavirus and enterobacterial agents, which have come to light as a result of recently developed immunologic techniques. The next section presents the nutritional consequences of acute diarrhea in children, progressing from the influence of diarrhea in the overall growth parameters in children to a discussion of the metabolic consequences of acute diarrhea, and then the exciting potential uses of bovine immunoglobulins for prevention. The following section includes an in-depth discussion of the effects of breast feeding on the nutritional status of infants. The reader will find the descriptions of infant breast feeding from the industrialized and the developing countries of the world to be especially interesting. The volume ends with a most timely review of the prospects for therapy and prevention. This section includes data describing the nutritional benefits related to oral therapy of acute diarrhea, a therapeutic intervention that has been introduced only in recent years. For those of us pediatricians trained in more traditional approaches of intravenous therapy, this section holds great fascination and interest. The volume concludes with a comprehensive review of newer vaccines that look promising for the prevention of acute diarrhea.

The workshop, which emanated from the International Center for Interdisciplinary Studies of Immunology at Georgetown University, also fulfills several of the objectives of the Center, including its mission of research, education, and patient care and its broader scope of community outreach and

technology transfer in areas that have international perspective as well as so-
cietal and ethical concerns and consequences.

The breadth of coverage of this volume should provide a book that will be
of interest to medical students, pediatricians, internists, general practitioners,
and nurses, as well as specialists in epidemiology, nutrition, microbiology,
immunology, and infectious diseases, and to all who are interested in improving the health of mothers and children throughout the world in order that
children might prosper on this earth.

Joseph A. Bellanti, M.D.
Washington, D.C.
January 1983

Foreword

Although still in its early stages, the Nestlé Nutrition Workshop Programme is already becoming an institution. Since the first workshop on maternal nutrition held in Rochegude, France, June 1980, under the chairmanship of Professor John Dobbing, Nestlé Nutrition has organized five other workshops and more are being planned.

All of the Nestlé Nutrition Workshops concentrate on pediatric nutrition, and this volume is the second in the series. Eventually, a new volume will be published every four months. The third book, *Nutritional Adaptation of the Gastrointestinal Tract*, is being edited by Professors A. Minkowski and N. Kretchmer. The fourth book will be *Iron Deficiency in Infancy and Childhood*, edited by Professor A. Stekel; the fifth will be *Human Milk Processing and the Nutrition of the Very Low Birthweight Infant* by Drs. J. D. Baum and A. F. Williams; and the sixth will be *Determinants in Infant Diarrhea Leading to Intractable Diarrhea and Infant Death*, edited by Professor E. Lebenthal.

By gathering together leading specialists on the chosen topics, we are confident that we are contributing to a better understanding of important problems in pediatric nutrition. We believe that these books will contribute to increased knowledge in pediatric nutrition as part of our commitment to assist in bringing about improved infant nutrition throughout the world.

P. R. Guesry, M.D.
Vice President
Nestlé Nutrition, S.A.

Acknowledgments

Many persons have contributed to the success of the workshop and to the preparation of this volume, and I wish to express my indebtedness to them. I first would like to thank Dr. Pierre R. Guesry, Medical and Scientific Director, Nestlé Nutrition, S.A., for his steadfast and encouraging support of the workshop from its inception to its completion, to Mr. Raphael Pagan and Dr. Thad M. Jackson of the Nestlé Coordination Center for Nutrition, Inc., for their great assistance in the preparation of the workshop and in the many details involved in organizing and accommodating an international meeting, and for Dr. E. De Maeyer's assistance in the preparation of the publication. I would like also to express my thanks to Mr. Edward Marasciulo and Dr. Jaimé C. Puccio of the Pan American Development Foundation for their advice and assistance in hosting the workshop. I would also like to express my appreciation to the Department of Pediatrics for their participation in the workshop and to Miss Barbara J. Claudy for her assistance, great diligence to detail and for her indefatigability in seeing the project through to its completion. Finally, I would like to express my sincere appreciation for the participation at the workshop of my first professor of pediatrics, Dr. Mitchell I. Rubin, who helped me see the vision of pediatrics and the values of the total approach to the child as a person.

Contents

Therapy and Prevention

Contributors

Stan Becker
International Centre for Diarrhoeal
*   Diseases Research*
Dacca, Bangladesh

Robert E. Black
Epidemiology Section
Center for Vaccine Development
University of Maryland
29 South Green Street
Baltimore, Maryland 21201

Kenneth H. Brown
Division of Human Nutrition
Department of International Health
Johns Hopkins University School of
*   Hygiene and Public Health*
Baltimore, Maryland 21205

R. K. Chandra
Department of Immunology
Janeway Child Health Centre
St. John's, Newfoundland, Canada

Robert Edelman
Clinical and Epidemiological Studies
*   Branch*
Microbiology and Infectious Diseases
*   Program*
National Institute of Allergy and
*   Infectious Diseases*
National Institutes of Health
Bethesda, Maryland 20205

H. Hilpert
Nestlé Research Laboratory
1800 Vevey, Switzerland

Rodrigo C. Hurtado
5597 Seminary Road
Baileys Crossroads, Virginia 22041

William J. Klish
Department of Pediatrics
Division of Pediatric Gastroenterology
*   and Nutrition*
University of Rochester Medical Center
Box 667
Rochester, New York 14627

Tasuke Konno
Department of Pediatrics
Tohoku University School of Medicine
Sendai 980, Japan

Frederick T. Koster
Department of Medicine
Division of Infectious Diseases
University of New Mexico
Albuquerque, New Mexico 87131

Toyoko Kutsuzawa
Department of Pediatrics
Tohoku University School of Medicine
Sendai 980, Japan

H. Link-Amster
Nestlé Research Laboratory
1800 Vevey, Switzerland

R. Lodinová-Žadníková
Research Institute for the Care of
*   Mother and Child*
Prague 4, Podolí, Czechoslovakia

Leonardo Mata
Instituto de Investigaciones en Salud
*   (INISA)*
Universidad de Costa Rica
Ciudad Universitaria Rodrigo Facio
San Pedro, Costa Rica

C. Mietens
*Westfälische Landeskinderklinik-
 Universitätsklinik und
Institut für Medizinische Mikrobiologie
 und Virologie der Ruhr-Universität
Bochum, West Germany*

José O. Mora
*Department of Community Medicine
Columbian School of Medicine
Calle 134, No. 13-81
Bogota, Columbia*

David R. Nalin
*Department of Epidemiology and
 Preventive Medicine
University of Maryland School of
 Medicine
10 South Pine Street
Baltimore, Maryland 20201*

Pearay L. Ogra
*Division of Infectious Diseases and
 Virology
Children's Hospital
Buffalo, New York 14222*

Marie Riepenhoff-Talty
*Division of Infectious Diseases and
 Virology
Children's Hospital
Buffalo, New York 14222*

Guillermo Ruiz-Palacios
*Infectious Disease Department
National Institute of Nutrition
Ave. San Fernando y Viaducto Tlalpan
Mexico 22, D.F., Mexico*

R. Bradley Sack
*Division of Geographic Medicine
The Johns Hopkins University School
 of Medicine
4940 Eastern Avenue
Baltimore, Maryland 21224*

M. Santosham
*Johns Hopkins Project
Box 1240
Whiteriver, Arizona 85941*

Benjamin José Schmidt
*Department of Pediatrics
Rua Cardoso de Almeida 2144
01251 Saõ Paulo, Brazil*

Hiroshi Suzuki
*Department of Pediatrics
Tohoku University School of Medicine
Sendai 980, Japan*

H. Tlaskalova-Hogenova
*Research Institute for the Care of
 Mother and Child
Prague 4, Podolí, Czechoslovakia*

H. Werchau
*Westfälische Landeskinderklinik-
 Universitätsklinik und
Institut für Medizinische Mikrobiologie
 und Virologie der Ruhr-Universität
Bochum, West Germany*

Robert H. Yolken
*Division of Infectious Diseases
Johns Hopkins University School of
 Medicine
600 North Wolfe Street
Baltimore, Maryland 21205*

Invited Attendees

Graeme Barnes/*Toronto, Canada*
Joseph A. Bellanti/*Washington, D.C.*
Carl Brandt/*Washington, D.C.*
Oscar Brunser/*Santiago, Chile*
Angel R. Colon/*Washington, D.C.*
Rodrigo Crespo/*Montevideo,
    Uruguay*
Delbert Dayton/*Bethesda, Maryland*
Carlos H. Daza/*Washington, D.C.*
Edouard De Maeyer/*Geneva,
    Switzerland*
Franklin de los Santos/*Montevideo,
    Uruguay*
Michael J. G. Farthing/*Boston,
    Massachusetts*
Lars A. Hanson/*Goteborg, Sweden*
Fr. Joseph Kadlec/*Washington, D.C.*
Samuel G. Kahn/*Washington, D.C.*
Albert Kapikian/*Bethesda, Maryland*
Gerald T. Keusch/*Boston,
    Massachusetts*

Emanuel Lebenthal/*Buffalo, New
    York*
Raul Leon Barua/*Lima, Peru*
Myron Levine/*Baltimore, Maryland*
Vijaya Melnick/*Bethesda, Maryland*
Sanford A. Miller/*Washington, D.C.*
Paul Offit/*Philadelphia, Pennsylvania*
Robert H. Parrott/*Washington, D.C.*
Nathaniel F. Pierce/*Baltimore,
    Maryland*
Jaimé C. Puccio/*Washington, D.C.*
John B. Robbins/*Bethesda,
    Maryland*
Mitchel I. Rubin/*Charleston, South
    Carolina*
Aderbal Sabra/*Rio de Janeiro, Brazil*
Humberto P. Soriano/*Santiago,
    Chile*
Robert M. Suskind/*Mobile, Alabama*
Raoul L. Wientzen/*Washington,
    D.C.*

Nestlé Participants

Pierre R. Guesry
*Vice President
Nestlé Nutrition, S.A.
1800 Vevey, Switzerland*

Thad Jackson
*Vice President
Nestlé Coordination Center for
    Nutrition, Inc.
1120 Connecticut Avenue, N.W.
Suite 310
Washington, D.C. 20036*

EPIDEMIOLOGY AND ETIOLOGY

Acute Diarrhea: Its Nutritional Consequences in Children, edited by J. A. Bellanti.
Nestlé, Vevey/Raven Press, New York © 1983.

EPIDEMIOLOGY OF ACUTE DIARRHEA IN CHILDHOOD

An Overview

Leonardo Mata

*Instituto de Investigaciones en Salud (INISA), Universidad de Costa Rica,
Ciudad Universitaria Rodrigo Facio, San Pedro, Costa Rica*

Much has been learned about the epidemiology of acute diarrheal disease since the folk conceptualization of a syndrome caused by "food indigestion." Despite early recognition of shigellosis, salmonellosis, giardiasis, and amebiasis as distinct clinical entities, there has been difficulty in the recent past in accepting that the remaining diarrheas were of an infectious nature. Furthermore, the appearance of diarrhea with the onset of weaning in many animal species and in man (18) and the systematic failure to find pathogenic agents in the majority of the diarrheas in the general population, contributed to questions of its infectious etiology.

However, epidemiologists, pediatricians, and microbiologists generally believed that the "nonspecific" diarrheas had a microbial or viral origin (16). The evidence was provided by field studies of diarrhea in urban and rural settings with low degrees of development. First, diarrhea is prevalent whenever sanitation and personal hygiene are deficient. Second, older persons are less frequently and less severely affected than infants and young children, indicating development of immunity. Third, in the community the epidemiology of acute diarrhea is similar to that of other infectious diseases, that is, secondary cases develop after contact with index cases, inducing self-limiting outbreaks or epidemics of varying magnitude. If personal hygiene and environmental sanitation are deficient, diarrhea becomes prevalent. Thus, it is easy to understand why morbidity and mortality rates due to diarrhea in developing nations today are, for instance, quite comparable to those of New York City at the turn of the century, when environmental conditions in New York at that time were as deficient as they are in most developing nations at present (25).

During the 1960s scientists were rewarded with the discovery of rotaviruses and "noncultivable" adenoviruses, and the rediscovery of other etiologic agents such as the enterotoxigenic Enterobacteriaceae, *Campylobacter*, *Yersinia*, and *Cryptosporidium* (ref. 37; see Table 1).

Bacterial colonization of the upper small intestine is common in rural children living under poor environmental conditions (19,23,33). It appears related to tropical jejunitis, chronic diarrhea, and malabsorption, which are so com-

TABLE 1. *Etiologic agents of human diarrhea*

Rotaviruses
Noncultivable adenoviruses
Cultivable adenoviruses
27 nm agents (Norwalk, Hawaii, Montgomery)
Enteroviruses (ECHO, coxsackie)
Coronaviruses
Astroviruses, calciviruses (?)

Enterotoxigenic *Escherichia coli* (ST, LT)
Enterophatogenic *Escherichia coli*
Enteroinvasive *Escherichia coli*
Shigella
Salmonella
Vibrio cholerae, other vibrios
Campylobacter fetus jejuni
Edwardsiella tarda
Yersinia enterocolitica
Aeromonas, Arizona, Plesiomonas

Entamoeba histolytica
Giardia lamblia
Dientamoeba fragilis
Balantidium coli
Isospora belli
Cryptosporidium

Trichuris trichiura
Strongyloides stercoralis
Hookworm
Trichinella spiralis
Capillaria philippinensis
Schistosoma mansoni

monly observed in developing countries. The phenomenon also occurs in adults who settle in tropical, unhygienic environments, to disappear upon return to a healthy setting (26). It is then possible that bacterial colonization of the upper small intestine, related to ingestion of contaminated water and foods, is causally associated with diarrhea and malabsorption. In this regard, weaning village foods have been found contaminated with fecal bacteria in different parts of the world (2,4,7).

Laboratory investigation reveals potential pathogens in about 60% of community diarrrhea cases, but many cases remain of unknown etiology ("nonspecific diarrheas") (Table 2). While technological advances in the last 15 years led to the discovery or recharacterization of such a variety of etiologic agents, one must consider the possibility that new viruses, new bacteria, new parasites, mycoplasmas, and chlamydia will be added to the list of agents of acute and chronic diarrhea in the human.

TRANSMISSION MECHANISMS

Transmission of diarrhea-causing agents is rather easy, since it involves a direct or indirect route from anus to mouth. The simplicity of the life cycle

TABLE 2. *Percent prevalence rates[a] of infectious agents in acute diarrhea seen at the hospital*

Agent	Dacca, Bangladesh (1979–1980)[b]	San José, Costa Rica (1976–1979)[c]
Enterotoxigenic *E. coli*	20.0	14.3
Rotaviruses	19.4	45.3
Shigella	11.6	8.1
C. fetus jejuni	11.6	8.0[d]
V. cholerae	5.5	not investigated
Nongroup 0:1 *Vibrio*	1.1	not investigated
Salmonella	0.6	7.3
E. histolytica	6.1	0
G. lamblia	5.6	4.5
No pathogen	17.6	36.8

[a] Rates of agents alone or combined with other(s).
[b] After ref. 55.
[c] After ref. 38.
[d] Survey in Dec. 1980–June 1981.

of most enteric protozoa, bacteria, and viruses, and the large number of infective units excreted in feces explain the high probability of transmission when personal hygiene and environmental sanitation are deficient. Contrary to other infectious agents that undergo some transformation in the outside environment before becoming infective for man, diarrhea-causing agents have the capacity to infect a new host without delay. Most agents are transmitted from person to person by direct contact through hands contaminated with feces, a common occurrence among children. Light clothing or nakedness and limited water availability are factors favoring this type of transmission in tropical and less developed areas. Feces disposed on the ground (especially in societies where indiscriminate squatting is the rule) are a source of contamination of foods and surface water, and of spreading by flies (60).

Pathogenic Enterobacteriaceae, *Campylobacter*, *Yersinia*, and *Cryptosporidium* in the human host have a zoonotic counterpart with similar infection patterns involving domestic animals. Animal rotaviruses, bacteria, and protozoa may induce diarrhea in man. Thus, transmission from animal to human has an epidemiology comparable to that described for person-to-person transmission.

DETERMINANTS OF INFECTION

Agent Determinants

Survival time in the environment of agents such as rotaviruses, 27 nm agents, and *Campylobacter* is not yet known, and information for other agents is limited (Table 3). Agents with a short survival time such as *Shigella* exhibit a high degree of communicability due to their greater virulence. Prevailing

TABLE 3. *Survival of diarrhea agents in the environment*

Less than 1 year
  Salmonella
  E. coli

Less than 6 months
  Giardia
  S. typhi
  Yersinia

Less than 1 month
  E. histolytica
  V. cholerae
  Shigella

Modified from ref. 60.

deficient host and environmental factors in less developed nations ensure successful transmission of most agents. On the other hand, improvement in environmental hygiene and education results in significant gains in prevention of infection.

Virulence is reflected in the infectious dose required for infection. This has been established experimentally for some pathogenic bacteria in well nourished adult volunteers (Table 4; refs. 11,60), but information may not be adequate for children, particularly when they are malnourished. The great number of virulent organisms excreted (see Table 4) ensures a good provision of the minimum infectious dose. Also, the dose required to induce diarrhea in adults probably is several hundred times greater than for children, as is the case of enteropathogenic *E. coli* (12). There are no data on the infectious dose of rotaviruses, adenoviruses, and 27 nm agents, or of *Campylobacter*, *Giardia*, and *Cryptosporidium*. This knowledge may have to await the development of suitable methods for isolating and growing some of these agents *in vitro*.

Host Determinants

Natural resistance depends on nonspecific resistance factors such as gastric acidity, intestinal motility, and indigenous microflora. A high concentration

TABLE 4. *Infectious dose of diarrhea agents in adult volunteers[a]*

Agent	Dose	Concentration/g feces
Shigella spp.	10^1–10^3	10^2–10^8
Salmonella spp.	10^5–10^8	10^2–10^8
Enterotoxigenic *E. coli*	10^8–10^{10}	10^4–10^9
V. cholerae	10^8–10^9	10^4–10^9

[a] Well nourished, American.
From ref. 60.

of hydrogen ions and digestive enzymes reduces microbial populations in ingested food and limits microbial growth in the intestinal milieu. Intestinal motility ensures a normal transit through the intestine, and therefore reduces opportunities for microbial multiplication (11). The intestinal microflora exerts inhibitory action toward pathogens, especially against bacteria, protozoa, and yeasts (11). The malnourished child may suffer from a decreased gastric acidity, a decreased intestinal motility, and a disturbed indigenous microbiota, allowing for adhesion, colonization, or invasion by diarrheal agents (35,53). Such alterations are particularly relevant in severe energy-protein malnutrition, but alterations in intestinal microflora are also observed following antibiotic treatment, an increasing problem in developing countries.

Breast-feeding provides a unique pool of nonspecific resistance factors, because colostrum and breast milk are rich in lactoferrin, lysozyme, complement and bifidus factors, lactoperoxydase, and interferon (15,41). These factors are present throughout all stages of lactation and exhibit great inhibitory or lytic capacity over most protozoa, bacteria, and viruses that infect and cause intestinal disease.

With regard to specific immunity, the dormant immune apparatus in the fetus becomes progressively competent after birth as the host encounters antigens, especially of microbial origin. The prominent immune cells, lymphocytes, are located in the thymus, spleen, intestine, bone marrow, blood, lymph glands, tonsils, appendix, and lamina propria. Cells in Peyer's patches effect intestinal immunity. Upon exposure to antigens, lymphocytes evolve and synthesize immunoglobulins. Specific IgM and secretory IgA are particularly relevant as they are effective against enteric agents in conjunction with complement and lysozyme. On the other hand, T lymphocytes in Peyer's patches, appendix, and other gut-associated lymphoid tissue (GALT) affect cellular immunity (11). Transformed T lymphocytes release lymphokines which are crucial in the elimination of the invading agent, an action carried out *in situ* or at a distance.

Specific immunity is also represented in human colostrum and milk. Specific antibodies to practically all enteric agents investigated have been recognized in human milk immunoglobulins, particularly in secretory IgA and in IgM. Immunoglobulin concentration and antibody titers are high in colostrum and decrease significantly in mature milk (61). However, the total amount of immunoglobulin remains high throughout lactation if the total volume of milk is taken into account. S-IgA is quite resistant to the action of gastric and intestinal enzymes as evidenced by its considerable activity upon recovery from feces (20). On the other hand, lymphocytes in human milk are functionally capable of effecting immune responses. Furthermore, lymphocytes homing towards the breast (10) may translocate and fall into the milk where specific activities can be observed (14). No changes in the quality and immune capacity of human milk appear to occur in undernourished women, although volume may be decreased. Chronic and acute malnutrition in children result in a marked reduction of the population of lymphoid cells, a notorious impairment of delayed hypersensitivity, and other expressions of cellular immunity (9). Nutritional recuperation leads to rapid correction of cellular immune deficiencies.

Host-Environment Determinants

Interactions between host and environment are the ultimate determinants of transmission and of the resulting epidemiological situation. The life cycle of enteric pathogens involves access of fecal bacteria to the mouth of susceptible individuals. The possible ways in which this is achieved depend on sociocultural characteristics of the population and the particular ecosystem in which it is settled. In prospective field studies conducted in Guatemala (28) and Bangladesh (1), it was found that both villages had a high rate of diarrheal disease with shigellosis as a prominent component (31,51). The epidemiology of diarrhea was very similar in both settings, with transmission further accentuated in Teknaff (Bangladesh) due to the observance of pardā (seclusion of women during child-bearing age) and ablution (washing of the opening of the urethra and anus after micturition and defecation) (1). It is easy to realize that transmission of diarrhea-causing agents is ultimately dependent on education, personal hygiene, and environmental sanitation, in sum, on socioeconomic development.

NATURAL HISTORY OF INTESTINAL INFECTION AND DIARRHEAL DISEASE

Colonization and Infection of Breast-Fed Children

Under normal conditions, the infant is born germ-free. Microbial colonization of the village newborn begins during passage through the birth canal and with exposure to maternal feces; within a few days, a predominant flora of gram-positive anaerobic bacilli develops, providing the infant is exclusively breast-fed (39). The hospital-born infant is more protected from fecal contamination, and the predominant intestinal microorganisms are gram-negative aerobic and anaerobic bacilli (54). Village newborns are exposed to enteric pathogens harbored by their mothers. Neonatal infection has been well documented in the village of Cauque (Table 5; ref. 28), but infections generally were spurious, transient, and asymptomatic, likely due to antiinfectious factors present in human colostrum and milk. Observation of maternal behavior, however, reveals that the newborn is not infrequently exposed to infectious agents as the mother often touches the child's mouth with her fingers. Furthermore, in every culture exclusively breast-fed infants are given small amounts of infusions, gruels, and other hand-prepared supplements that can be easily contaminated (28).

TABLE 5. *Frequency of enteric infections among mothers and neonates[a]*

Agent	Percent
Mothers	
Enteroviruses	25
Shigella	9
Salmonella	5
E. histolytica	54
Giardia	8
Ascaris	83
Neonates	
Enteroviruses, 3rd day	3.7
Shigella, 2nd–4th week	3.6
Protozoa, 1st week	5

[a] Cauqué, 1964–1969.

The remarkable protection afforded by maternal milk is observed in the low rate of acquisition of *Shigella* and *Giardia* during exclusive breast-feeding. Prospective studies in Cauqué revealed that infants are quite refractory to these agents during the first 6 to 9 months of life (Fig. 1). Consumption of contaminated foods increases with weaning, as protection from human milk decreases; then infection with pathogens becomes prominent. This does not necessarily apply to infants living in environments with good sanitation.

Role of Weaning Foods

Contaminated fingers, utensils, and foods play an important role in the epidemiology of diarrhea. Weaning foods were previously neglected, but ob-

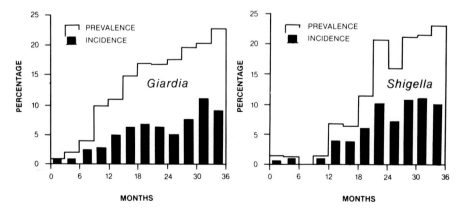

FIG. 1. Incidence and prevalence of *Giardia* and *Shigella* infections in a cohort of 45 Mayan Indian children in Santa Maria Cauqué, observed from birth to 3 years of age (1964–1969). Rates were calculated from weekly examinations (*Giardia*) or cultures (*Shigella*) of feces. (After ref. 40.)

TABLE 6. *Fecal bacteria and other potential enteric pathogens in village weaning foods*

Country	Food	Bacteria, $\log_{10}$/g or ml
Guatemala[a] (Cauqué)	Tortillas	E. coli, 3–7 S. aureus, 7–8 B. cereus, 9 Clostridium sp., 1–2
Gambia[b] (Keneba)	Cereal gruels, milk	E. coli, > 5 S. aureus, 2–6 B. cereus, 4–6 C. welchii, 3–5
Bangladesh[c] (Matlab)	Rice, milk	E. coli, 2–7

[a] From ref. 7.
[b] From ref. 2.
[c] From ref. 4.

servations in Guatemala showed that fecal bacteria and other potential pathogens such as *Bacillus cereus* proliferate in tortillas stored under usual village conditions (7). In The Gambia and Bangladesh, weaning foods also carry enteric bacteria (Table 6; refs. 2, 4). Contamination of weaning foods increases during the rainy and warm months when conditions within the home favor multiplication of microorganisms in food (4), thus accounting for part of the seasonality of bacterial diarrhea.

INCIDENCE OF DIARRHEAL DISEASE

Intensive surveillance involving more than one visit per week to Cauqué homes showed a rate of 792 diarrhea cases per 100 person-years, which is

TABLE 7. *Diarrhea, dysentery, and certain symptoms in 45 cohort children observed from birth to age 3 years[a]*

Observations	No. of episodes	% All illnesses	Rate/100 person-years	Mean events/ child/year
Illness				
Diarrhea	953	38.93	719.2	7.2
Dysentery	97	3.96	73.2	0.7
Total	1,050	42.89	792.4	7.9
Symptom				
Fever, $\geq 37.5°C$	1,148		873.0	8.7
Vomiting	235		178.7	1.8
Anorexia	823		625.8	6.3

[a] Santa Maria Cauqué, 1964–1969.
Adapted from ref. 28.

TABLE 8. *Incidence of common infectious diseases per 100 person-months[a]*

Illness	Age (months)					
	0–5	6–11	12–17	18–23	24–29	30–35
	270[b]	270	270	270	255	250
Diarrhea	33.3	63.0	77.8	87.4	78.0	55.0
Upper respiratory	25.6	34.1	33.3	31.1	30.1	35.7
Lower respiratory	15.9	23.0	23.7	27.4	24.3	14.0
Eye	21.9	18.5	13.7	14.4	8.9	5.0
Mouth	9.3	6.3	8.2	4.1	7.0	3.9
Skin, scalp	1.9	3.3	2.2	6.3	2.7	4.7
Common communicable	1.9	10.0	8.2	9.6	7.7	7.4
Other[c]	0.7	1.1	2.2	4.1	1.2	1.9
Ear	0.7	0.4	1.5	0.4	1.9	0.8
Total	111.1	159.7	170.7	184.8	161.8	128.3

[a] Forty-five Cauqué children observed from birth to 3 years of age (1964–1969).
[b] Number of person-months.
[c] Genitourinary tract; fevers; ringworm; tenosynovitis.
From ref. 39.

equivalent to 7.9 cases per child per year (Table 7). High incidence rates of fever, vomiting, anorexia, and dehydration were recorded (Table 8; ref. 28). These data depart from those of other rural studies which revealed about two diarrhea episodes per child per year (18,52,53). Differences in definition of diarrhea and in intensity of surveillance could explain the noted discrepancies; recent observations in Matlab, Bangladesh (5) showed figures similar to those in Cauqué.

Age Distribution

Infection during the first 3 years of life is age-dependent, as illustrated with *Shigella* in a prospective observation of 45 cohort children (Figs. 1, 2). Differences in occurrence of serotypes occurred throughout 6 years of observation (from the year of birth of the first cohort child to the year the last cohort child was 3 years old), revealing a very low prevalence in the first 2 years while the cohort was barely 1 year old. Distinct outbreaks of various *Shigella* serotypes occurred in certain years (Fig. 3; ref. 28).

The pattern of infection with parasites, enteroviruses, and cultivable adenoviruses was similar; their frequency increased with age, reaching the highest incidence and prevalence at the peak of weaning and in the following months (28). Obviously, diarrheal disease showed a similar age distribution (Table 8; Fig. 4), their frequency increasing after the first 6 months of life and reaching a peak at weaning, around 18 months in the study village. Thereafter, the frequency of diarrheal disease tended to diminish although rates were persistently high throughout preschool age. In societies where children are weaned in the first year of life, the peak of diarrhea occurs in that year.

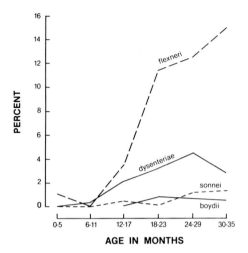

FIG. 2. Prevalence (percentage) of *Shigella* cases and carriers, by age, in a cohort of 45 Mayan Indian children, observed from birth to 3 years of age (1964–1969). (From ref. 28.)

Seasonality

The recent recognition of rotaviruses and enterotoxigenic bacteria has enabled a better characterization of the seasonality of diarrhea. In developing countries, the bulk of diarrhea occurs during the hot, humid, and rainy season,

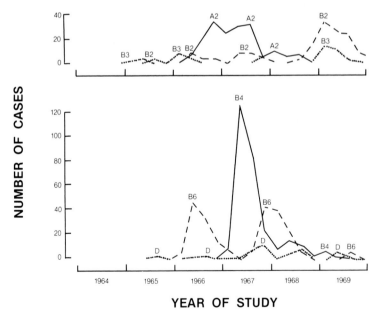

FIG. 3. Outbreaks of *Shigella* cases and carriers in a cohort of 45 Mayan Indian children observed from birth to 3 years of age (1964–1969). Few shigellae were isolated during the first year of life; as the cohort aged, infections increased. Outbreaks of *S. flexneri 4, S. flexneri 6, S. dysenteriae 2,* and *S. flexneri 2* were, in that order, more prominent. (From ref. 28.)

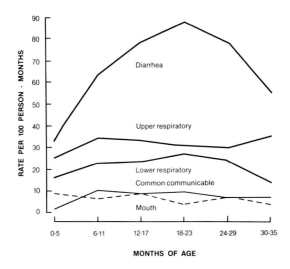

FIG. 4. Incidence of infectious diseases, Santa Maria Cauqué (1964–1969).

and is generally associated with enterotoxigenic bacteria, *Shigella*, and other bacteria (6,38). During this season there is an apparent increase in bacterial contamination of water and village foods (4). On the other hand, rotaviruses are more frequent in the dry, cold season, especially in countries with temperate climate (13,22,24). As nations move from a traditional to a modern way of life, the "winter" viral diarrhea peak becomes increasingly prominent, and the "summer" bacterial diarrhea season decreases in importance. The significance of seasonality in diarrhea cannot be ignored as it is one of the factors determining rural poverty (8). Seasonal variation may be aggravated by the appearance of unusually virulent strains that may induce community epidemics lasting for months or even years (17).

NUTRITIONAL IMPLICATIONS OF DIARRHEA

Anorexia is a frequent symptom of diarrhea, resulting in significant reductions in food intake (34,35,58). A protein-losing enteropathy occurs in diarrheas due to tissue-invading bacteria and viruses (57). Alterations in absorption occur in diarrheas of various etiologies (44). Furthermore, diarrheas cause wastage and stunting (32,35).

These observations have led to a greater recognition of diarrhea as a malnourishing factor. A considerable proportion of the malnutrition observed in the community results from recurrent enteric infection. Diarrhea is a frequent precipitating factor of marasmus and kwashiorkor, especially where weaning occurs during the second or third year of life; diarrhea leads to marasmus when weaning is effected prematurely in the first year of life.

TABLE 9. *Comparison of diarrheal disease mortality in the Americas[a]*

Region	Age (years)			
	< 1		1–4	
	Rate	%	Rate	%
North	19	1.4	0.6	0.9
Caribbean	439	15.2	28	15.0
Central	1,078	22.8	154	25.8
South, tropical	1,066	20.3	151	21.5
South, temperate	496	10.9	20	9.1

[a] Rates per 100,000 and proportionate mortality (1976).
Adapted from ref. 47.

MORTALITY DUE TO DIARRHEAL DISEASE

Despite great difficulties in obtaining statistics on diarrhea deaths in many developing nations, reliable data for 1976 was available from the Pan American Health Organization (PAHO) (47). Striking differences are noted between rates in North America and Tropical America (Mexico, Central America, the Caribbean, and Tropical South America) (Table 9). In Tropical America, diarrhea accounted for 15 to 23% of all infant deaths, and for 15 to 26% of deaths in preschool children. Diarrhea was the leading cause of death in at least five countries, and the second cause in another ten countries. On the basis of an observed two cases of diarrhea per child per year (2a), it can be estimated that 100 million cases with 100,000 deaths would have occurred in Latin America in 1976. If seven to eight diarrhea episodes per child per year are considered (28), the estimated diarrhea cases in Latin America in 1976 were 350 million.

Secular changes in mortality have been documented in less developed countries throughout the world (45); this is probably due to the dissemination of health information and to improvements in the quality of life. Figure 5 illustrates differences in diarrheal disease death rates for infants and preschool children in American nations during the period 1973 to 1977 (47).

Figure 6 shows mean annual percent variation in diarrhea death rates within the 1968 to 1977 period (47). Countries arranged by decreasing magnitude of mean annual percent variations show that Dominica had the greatest improvement, as diarrhea decreased at a velocity of 13.8% per year (infants) and 15.6% per year (preschool children). In general, trends for infants and preschool children changed in a similar fashion in most countries. The nations doing better during the period investigated were—in addition to Dominica—Costa Rica, Dominican Republic, Chile, and Mexico. Venezuela showed only a small improvement, whereas Ecuador and El Salvador actually had an increase in mortality rate. The cases of Trinidad-Tobago and Barbados deserve special mention because the health situation in these islands is relatively good, yet

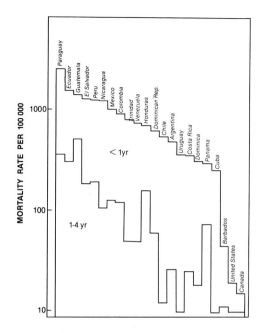

FIG. 5. Diarrheal mortality in the Americas, children 0–4 years (1973–1977).

mortality has increased; it may be helpful to find out if changes in notification and recording of diarrhea deaths occurred in these countries during the study period. In general, the data should bring optimism inasmuch as they reflect an overall improvement in the quality of life in many Latin American nations in recent years.

CORRELATION OF DIARRHEA MORTALITY AND INFANT MORTALITY RATES

Diarrheal disease is one of the main determinants of early death, although the mechanism is not totally understood. The risk of death increases when malnutrition is present, but well nourished individuals may also die, partic-

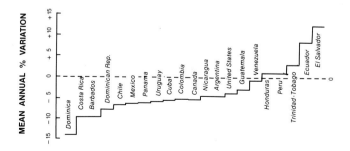

FIG. 6. Annual percent variation in diarrheal mortality (1968–1977).

ularly during epidemics of highly virulent organisms such as the Shiga bacillus (42). Artificially fed infants are the most susceptible to die from diarrhea; weaned neonates who develop diarrhea are prone to dehydrate and succumb if they are not rapidly rehydrated (49).

Diarrheal disease accounts for as much as 30% of all infant deaths in some developing countries; a high correlation between infant and diarrheal mortality is then expected. Adequate diarrhea mortality figures are available for Costa Rica from 1926 onwards; they reveal a rapid decline in mortality particularly in recent years (Fig. 7). After a period of slow decrease in mortalities that ended around 1940, an abrupt decline took place coinciding with social reforms in the country. Civil strife, migration, population increase, and shift to bottle-feeding coincided with stagnation in rates lasting until about the 1960s. Thereafter, diarrhea death-rates declined dramatically to reach 4.5 per 100,000 in 1981. The profiles of infant and diarrheal disease mortality matched year by year (Fig. 8). The main correspondence was observed with postneonatal infant mortality, and less with the neonatal rates (30,35). A significant correlation was noted from 1942 onwards, indicating that diarrheal disease mortality is a determinant of infant death. The striking changes in health in Costa Rica in the last 15 years are in accord with the gains in social justice, literacy, environmental sanitation (especially water supply), and income, all occurring within a frame of peace and democracy (36,43). The improvements went together with a strengthening of the health infrastructure culminating in a decade of programs and expansion of health interventions, particularly in the rural area (43,56). Intradomiciliary potable water supply, for example, was

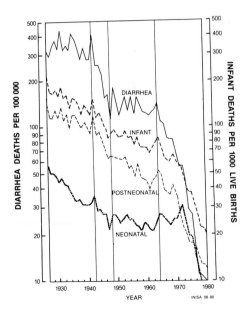

FIG. 7. Infant and diarrheal mortality in Costa Rica during the period 1930–1980.

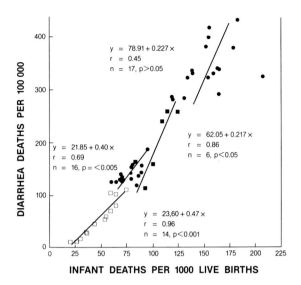

FIG. 8. Correlation between infant mortality and diarrheal disease death rates in Costa Rica (1926–1978). Numbers next to *data points* indicate the year of the correlated indexes. Correlations were significant for the entire period, except for 1926–1942. Underreporting in 1926 and 1927 probably accounted for lower death rates and this influenced the correlation (30).

available in 1980 to 70% of the sparse rural population, illiteracy rate was about 12%, and income was $1,800 per capita.

DISCUSSION

The most important issue of diarrheal diseases concerns their control and prevention. The history of industrialized nations shows that the control and prevention of diarrhea rests on an improvement in the whole environment. This also appears to be the case in some developing countries such as Cuba and Costa Rica.

On the other hand, oral rehydration (59) and breast-feeding (21,29) are of great value in the struggle against diarrhea. Oral rehydration is of particular interest when applied to rural situations, as shown in the Philippines, Turkey, Bangladesh, Egypt, and other nations (48). Free distribution of oral rehydration salts (ORS) in Bangladesh in a population where diarrheal disease is highly endemic resulted in a drastic decline in mortality (Table 10; ref. 50). In 1978, an aggressive program of oral rehydration was started at the National Children's Hospital (Costa Rica), resulting in a decrease in diarrhea lethality of more than 90% (Table 11; ref. 46). An oral rehydration program for the general population was then initiated in Costa Rica in 1980, with distribution of free ORS sachets to all health centers and posts. The program was expanded to include more

TABLE 10. *Effect of oral rehydration on rural mortality[a]*

Age (years)	% Case fatality		Mortality per 1,000	
	Shamlapur	Controls	Shamlapur	Controls
< 1	0.5	6.3	1.6	17.4
1–4	0.9	2.3	1.9	5.7
5–9	0.4	1.3	0.4	1.3
10+	0.2	1.7	0.2	1.4
Total	0.5	2.4	0.6	2.9

[a] Shamlapur, Bangladesh.
From ref. 50.

than 200,000 homes (27), and has contributed to the gains observed in childhood mortality in the last 2 years (see Fig. 7).

Another avenue for control and prevention relates to breast-feeding in view of its health promotion capacity (21,29). This is particularly important in less-developed countries where the environment provides ample opportunities for continuous intestinal infection of toddlers. Breast-feeding is equally important in transitional societies as they experience a decline in breast-feeding as part of the westernization process. In an ongoing long-term prospective study in the transitional population of Puriscal, Costa Rica, mother–infant interaction, rooming-in, and other means of promoting breast-feeding were implemented in the gynecoobstetric service. Prospective observation of the population revealed that breast-feeding became almost universal from a previous 25% failure to breast-feed and 30% weaning in the first months of life (32). A significantly lower incidence of diarrheal disease was recorded among the exclusively breast-fed than in the supplemented infants (Table 12). Also, these had less diarrhea than the completely weaned infants, up to the age of 6 months. Thereafter, there were no significant differences between breast-fed and weaned infants, but it must be kept in mind that the quality of life in this transitional population is much better than in most traditional societies.

Regarding other approaches toward control and prevention of acute diarrhea, the development of antirotavirus and antienterotoxin *E. coli* vaccines

TABLE 11. *Diarrhea lethality[a]*

Year	Cases	Deaths[b]	Lethality per 1,000	Rehydration route	% Reduction
1977	5,974	18	3.0	Slow i.v.	
1978	6,000	2	0.3	Oral (90%) Rapid i.v. (10%)	90

[a] National Children's Hospital, Costa Rica, 1977–1978.
[b] After 48 hr internment.
Adapted from ref. 46.

TABLE 12. Incidence of diarrheal disease by age and feeding regime in 577 cohort rural infants[a]

Age (months)	Breast-fed				Non-breast-fed	
	Exclusively		Supplemented			
	Infants (p-m)[b]	Diarrheas (rate/100 p-m)	Infants (p-m)	Diarrheas (rate/100 p-m)	Infants (p-m)	Diarrheas (rate/100 p-m)
0–2	350 (1,050)	20 (1.9)[c]	181 (543)	14 (2.6)	46 (138)	17 (12.3)
3–5	50 (150)	2 (0.7)	365 (1,095)	47 (4.3)	159 (477)	43 (9.0)
6–8	0		2,922 (876)	45 (5.1)	349 (1,047)	69 (6.6)
9–11	0		222 (666)	39 (5.8)	349 (1,047)	62 (5.9)

[a] Puriscal, Costa Rica, 1979–1982.
[b] p-m = person-months of experience, obtained by multiplying the number of infants by the number of months in each period.
[c] An attack rate of 1.9 per 100 p-m is equivalent to 5.7 cases per 100 infants in the 0–2 month period, or to 0.057 cases per child in the first 3 months of life.

is investigated at the present time, though tangible results may be far away. The ultimate control and prevention lie in an overall improvement of personal hygiene, water supply, food hygiene, waste disposal, and so forth. Such change demands a holistic approach focusing on improving education, income, environmental sanitation, child care practices, and health services (28).

The recent examples of Costa Rica, Cuba, and some other poor nations, point toward the importance of improving the quality of life as the ultimate goal in public health practice compatible with the fundamental rights of the human society.

REFERENCES

1. Aziz, K. M. A., Hasan, K. Z., Patwary, Y. et al. (1981): A study of interpersonal spread of human faeces in rural Teknaff of Bangladesh. *ICDDR,B.*, Dacca.
2. Barrell, R. A. E., and Rowland, M. G. M. (1979): Infant foods as a potential source of diarrhoeal illness in rural West Africa. *Trans. R. Soc. Trop. Med. Hyg.*, 73:85–90.
2a. Barua, D. (1981): Diarrhea as a global problem and the WHO programme for its control. In: *Acute Enteric Infections in Children. New Prospects for Treatment and Prevention*, edited by T. Holme, J. Holmgren, M. H. Merson, and R. Mollby, pp. 1–6. Elsevier/North Holland, Amsterdam.
3. Black, R. E., Brown, K. H., and Becker, S. (1982): Comments on overview of acute diarrhea in children. *Conference on Acute Diarrhea: Its Nutritional Consequences in Children*. Georgetown University, Washington, D.C.
4. Black, R. E., Brown, K. H., Becker, S. et al. (1982): Contamination of weaning foods and transmission of enterotoxigenic *Escherichia coli* diarrhoea in children in rural Bangladesh. *Trans. R. Soc. Trop. Med. Hyg.* (*in press*).
5. Black, R. E., Brown, K. H., Becker, S., and Yanus, M. (1982): Longitudinal studies of infectious diseases and physical growth of children in rural Bangladesh. I. Patterns of morbidity. *Am. J. Epidemiol.*, 115:305–314.
6. Black, R. E., Merson, M. H., Rahman, A. S. M. M., et al. (1980): *J. Infect. Dis.*, 142:660–664.
7. Capparelli, E., and Mata, L. (1975): Microflora of maize prepared as tortillas. *Appl. Microbiol.*, 29:802–806.
8. Chambers, R., Longhurst, R., Bradley, D., and Feachem, R. (1979): *Seasonal Dimensions to Rural Poverty: Analysis and Practical Implications*. Institute of Developmental Studies, University of Sussex, Brighton, England, p. 28.
9. Chandra, R. K., and Newberne, P. M. (1977): *Nutrition, Immunity and Infection. Mechanisms of Interactions*. Plenum Press, New York.
10. Craig, S. W., Cebra, J. J. (1971): Peyer's patches: an enriched source of precursors for IgA-producing immunocytes in the rabbit. *J. Exp. Med.*, 134:188–200.
11. DuPont, H. L., and Pickering, L. K. (1980): *Infections of the Gastrointestinal Tract. Microbiology, Pathophysiology and Clinical Features*. Plenum, New York.
12. Ferguson, W. W., and June, R. C. (1952): Experiments on feeding adult volunteers with *Escherichia coli* 111, B4, a coliform organism associated with infant diarrhea. *Am. J. Hyg.*, 55:155–169.
13. Flewett, T. H., Bryden, A. S., and Davies, H. (1974): Diagnostic electron microscopy of faeces. I. The viral flora of the faeces as seen by electron microscopy. *J. Clin. Pathol.*, 27:603–614.
14. Goldblum, R. M., Ahlstedt, B., Carlsson, L. et al. (1975): Antibody-forming cells in human colostrum after oral immunization. *Nature*, 257:797–798.
15. Goldman, A. S., and Smith, C. W. (1973): Host resistance factors in human milk. *J. Pediatr.*, 82:1082–1090.
16. Gordon, J. E. (1964): Acute diarrheal disease. *Am. J. Med. Sci.*, 248:345–365.
17. Gordon, J. E., Ascoli, W., Pierce, V., et al. (1965): Studies of diarrheal disease in Central America. VI. An epidemic of diarrhea in a Guatemalan highland village, with a component due to *Shigella dysenteriae*, type 1. *Am. J. Trop. Med. Hyg.*, 14:404–411.

18. Gordon, J. E., Chitkara, I. D., and Wyon, J. B. (1963): Weanling diarrhea. *Am. J. Med. Sci.*, 245:345–377.
19. Gracey, M. S. (1979): The contaminated small bowel syndrome. *Am. J. Clin. Nutr.*, 32:234–243.
20. Hanson, L. A., Carlsson, B., Ahlstedt, S. et al. (1975): Immune defense factors in human milk. *Mod. Probl. Paediatr.*, 15:63–72.
21. Jelliffe, D. B., and Jelliffe, E. F. P. (1978): *Human Milk in the Modern World. Psychological, Nutritional and Economic Significance.* Oxford University Press, New York.
22. Kapikian, A. Z., Kim, H. W., Wyatt, R. G. et al. (1978): Human reovirus-like agent as the major pathogen associated with "winter" gastroenteritis in hospitalized infants and young children. *N. Engl. J. Med.*, 294:965–972.
23. Klipstein, F. A., Short, H. B., Engert, R. F. et al. (1976): Contamination of the small intestine by enterotoxigenic coliform bacteria among the rural population of Haiti. *Gastroenterology*, 70:1035–1041.
24. Konno, T., Suzuki, H., Imai, A. et al. (1978): A long-term survey of rotavirus infection in Japanese children with acute gastroenteritis. *J. Infect. Dis.*, 138:569–576.
25. Levine, M. M., and Edelman, R. (1979): Acute diarrheal infections in infants. I. Epidemiology, treatment, and prospects for immunoprophylaxis. *Hosp. Pract.*, 14:89–100.
26. Lindebaum, J., Gerson, C. D., and Kent, T. H. (1971): Recovery of small-intestinal structure and function after residence in the tropics. I. Studies in Peace Corps volunteers. *Ann. Int. Med.*, 74:218–222.
27. López, M. E., and Hidalgo, M. A. (1981): Diarrhea control program in Costa Rica. In: *International Workshop on Planning and Management of National Programs of Diarrheal Disease Control*, PAHO, Honduras.
28. Mata, L. J. (1978): *The Children of Santa María Cauqué. A Prospective Field Study of Health and Growth.* MIT Press, Cambridge.
29. Mata, L. (1978): Breast-feeding: main promoter of infant health. *Am. J. Clin. Nutr.*, 31:2058–2065.
30. Mata, L. (1981): Epidemiologic perspective of diarrheal disease in Costa Rica and current efforts in control, prevention and research. *Rev. Lat.-Am. Microbiol.*, 23:109–119.
31. Mata, L. J., Fernández, R., and Urrutia, J. J. (1969): Infección del intestino por bacterias enteropatógenas en niños de una aldea de Guatemala, durante los tres primeros años de vida. *Rev. Lat.-Am. Microbiol. Parasitol.*, 11:102–109.
32. Mata, L., Jiménez, P., Allen, M. A. et al. (1981): Diarrhea and malnutrition: breast-feeding intervention in a transitional population. In: *Acute Enteric Infections in Children. New Prospects for Treatment and Prevention*, pp. 233–251. Elsevier/North-Holland, Amsterdam.
33. Mata, L. J., Jiménez, F., Cordón, M. et al. (1972): Gastrointestinal flora of children with protein-calorie malnutrition. *Am. J. Clin. Nutr.*, 25:1118–1126.
34. Mata, L. J., Kronmal, R. A., Urrutia, J. J., and García, B. (1977): Effect of infection on food intake and the nutritional state: perspectives as viewed from the village. *Am. J. Clin. Nutr.*, 30:1215–1227.
35. Mata, L., Kronmal, R. A., and Villegas, H. (1980): Diarrheal diseases: A leading world health problem. In: *Cholera and Related Diarrheas*, 43rd Nobel Symposium, pp. 1–14. Karger, Basel.
36. Mata, L., and Mohs, E. (1978): As seen from national levels: developing world. In: *Progress in Human Nutrition*, Vol. 2, pp. 254–264, Ari, Westport, Connecticut.
37. Mata, L., and Simhon, A. (1982): Enteritis y colitis infecciosa del hombre. *Adel. Microbiol. Enf. Infecc.*, 1:1–50.
38. Mata, L., Simhon, A., Padilla, R. et al. (1983): Diarrhea associated with rotaviruses, enterotoxigenic *Escherichia coli, Campylobacter* and other agents in Costa Rican children, 1976–1981. *Am. J. Trop. Med. Hyg.*, 32:146–153.
39. Mata, L. J., and Urrutia, J. J. (1971): Intestinal colonization of breast-fed children in a rural area of low socioeconomic level. *Ann. NY Acad. Sci.*, 176:93–109.
40. Mata, L. J., Urrutia, J. J., Cáceres, A., and Guzmán, M. A. (1972): The biological environment in a Guatemalan rural community. In: *Proceedings Western Hemisphere Nutrition Congress III*, pp. 257–264. Futura, New York.
41. Mata, L. J., and Wyatt, R. G. (1971): The uniqueness of human milk. Host resistance to infection. *Am. J. Clin. Nutr.*, 24:976–986.
42. Mendizábal-Morris, C. A., Mata, L. J., Gangarosa, L., and Guzmán, G. (1971): Epidemic

Shiga dysentery in Central America. II. Magnitude of the outbreak and mortality in Guatemala in 1969. *Am. J. Trop. Med. Hyg.*, 20:927–933.
43. Mohs, E. (1980): *Salud y Democracia. El Surgimiento de una Nueva Era.* Escuela Med., Univ. Costa Rica.
44. Molla, A., Molla, A. M., Sarker, S. A. et al. (1981): Effects of diarrhoea on absorption of macronutrients during acute stage and recovery. ICDDR,B., Working Paper No. 19, Dacca.
45. Nájera, E. (1976): Socioepidemiología de las enfermedades diarreicas agudas, incluido el cólera. *Rev. Sanid. Hig. Pública*, 50:5–77.
46. Odio, C., and Mohs, E. (1980): Características actuales de la letalidad por diarrea. *Rev. Méd. Hosp. Nac. Niños (Costa Rica)*, 15:181–187.
47. Pan American Health Organization (PAHO) (1980): Enfermedades diarreicas en las Américas. *Bol. Epidemiol. (PAHO)*, 1:1–4.
48. Parker, R. L., Rinehart, W., Piotrow, P. T., and Doucette, L. (1981): La terapia de rehidratación oral (TRO) en el tratamiento de la diarrea infantil. *Popul. Rep.*, Series L(2):1–41.
49. Pizarro, D., Posada, G., Mata, L. et al. (1979): Oral rehydration of neonates with dehydration diarrhoeas. *Lancet*, 2:1209–1210.
50. Rahaman, M. M., Aziz, K. M. S., Patwari, Y., and Munshi, M. H. (1979): Diarrhoeal mortality in two Bangladeshi villages with and without community-based oral rehydration therapy. *Lancet*, 2:809–812.
51. Rahaman, M. M., Khan, M. M., Aziz, K. M. S. et al. (1975): An outbreak of dysentery caused by *Shigella dysenteriae* type 1 on a coral island in the Bay of Bengal. *J. Infect. Dis.*, 132:15–19.
52. Rohde, J. E., and Northrup, R. S. (1976): Taking science where the diarrhea is. In: *Acute Diarrhoea in Childhood*, Ciba Foundation Symposium No. 42 (new series), pp. 339–358. Elsevier, Excerpta Medica, North-Holland, Amsterdam.
53. Scrimshaw, N. S., Taylor, C. E., and Gordon, J. E. (1968): *Interactions of Nutrition and Infection.* WHO Monograph No. 57, Geneva.
54. Simhon, A., Douglas, J. R., Drasar, B. S., and Soothill, J. F. (1982): Effect of feeding on infants' faecal flora. *Arch. Dis. Child.*, 57:54–58.
55. Stoll, B. J., Glass, R. I., Hug, M. I., et al. (1982): Surveillance of patients attending a diarrheal disease hospital in Bangladesh. *J. Infect. Dis.*, 146:177–183.
56. Villegas, H., and Osuna, J. (1979): Extensión de los servicios de salud de Costa Rica. In: *Condiciones de Salud del Niño en las Américas.* PAHO, No. 381, pp. 168–183.
57. Wahed, M. A., Rahaman, M. M., Gilman, R. H. et al. (1981): Protein-losing enteropathy in diarrhoea: application of α_1-antitrypsin assay. *ICDDR,B.*, Working Paper No. 22. Dacca.
58. Whitehead, R. G. (1981): Malnutrition and infection. In: *The Impact of Malnutrition on Immune Defense in Parasitic Infestation*, pp. 15–25. Hans Huber, Bern.
59. World Health Organization (WHO) (1977): A positive effect on the nutrition of Philippine children of an oral glucose-electrolyte solution given at home for the treatment of diarrhoea. Report of a field trial by an international study group. *Bull. WHO*, 55:87–94.
60. World Health Organization (WHO) (1980): *Environmental Health and Diarrhoeal Disease Prevention.* WHO/DDC/80.5, Geneva.
61. Wyatt, R. G., García, B., Cáceres, A., and Mata, L. J. (1972): Immunoglobulins and antibodies in colostrum and milk of Guatemalan Mayan women. *Arch. Latinoam. Nutr.*, 22:629–644.

Acute Diarrhea: Its Nutritional Consequences in Children, edited by J. A. Bellanti.
Nestlé, Vevey/Raven Press, New York © 1983.

Epidemiology of Acute Diarrhea in Childhood

Comments

*†Robert E. Black, *‡Kenneth H. Brown, and *Stan Becker

*International Centre for Diarrhoeal Diseases Research, Dacca, Bangladesh; †Center for Vaccine Development, University of Maryland School of Medicine, Baltimore, Maryland 21201; and ‡Division of Human Nutrition, Department of International Health, Johns Hopkins University School of Hygiene and Public Health, Baltimore, Maryland 21205

During studies in the 1950s and 1960s, investigators recognized the importance of the diarrheal diseases that occur when infants are shifted from exclusive breast-feeding to a mixed diet (5,7). The recognition of this "weaning diarrhea" has focused attention on the causes and prevention of diarrhea during this critical period in the infant's life.

Several studies have demonstrated a lower incidence of diarrhea in breast-fed infants than in partially breast-fed or in artificially fed infants during the first few months of life (4,8). This may be because of protective factors in breast milk, such as leucocytes, specific immunoglobulins, and nonspecific antiinfectious factors (9); however, an equal, if not more important, protective feature of exclusive breast-feeding is that infants avoid ingesting contaminated foods. Thus, many public health workers have advocated programs emphasizing that infants can be exclusively breast-fed for at least the first 3 to 6 months, and investigators, such as Dr. L. Mata, have paved the way with innovative programs, such as the one in Puriscal, to promote breast-feeding (6). It is likely that such efforts will reduce the incidence and severity of diarrhea during the time that infants are exclusively breast-fed, but it is also likely that diarrhea rates will increase when complementary foods are eventually introduced. To take specific measures to prevent diarrhea, it is necessary to have a better understanding of the role of food and water contamination in the transmission of the various enteropathogens in infants.

The hazard of contamination of milk given to bottle-fed babies has received a great deal of attention and deserves emphasis, particularly in urban and peri-urban areas of developing countries. However, many of the children suffering from high rates of diarrhea in developing countries are breast-fed and given traditional weaning foods, such as starchy pastes made with rice, maize, potato, wheat, banana, or other locally available foods; animal milk may also be given. Studies in The Gambia demonstrated that these foods can be as hazardous, bacteriologically, as bottle formulae when prepared in the usual unhygienic home environments of rural villages (1). In addition, these studies showed that the level of contamination was related to the time of storage of the food at ambient temperature, presumably because of bacterial multiplication in the food.

Our studies of two rural communities in Bangladesh provided an opportunity to measure the degree of bacterial contamination of traditional weaning foods and to determine if these foods could be directly implicated in the transmission of diarrheal diseases. As part of longitudinal studies of a cohort of children, dietary intake was determined monthly for 1 year in 70 children, 5 to 18 months old at the beginning of the study (3). All foods consumed by children on the days of study were weighed and samples of food and water were taken for bacteriological study (2).

In this area, breast-feeding was universally initiated and continued for 2 to 3 years (3). At 12 months of age, all infants were still receiving breast milk and consuming about 600 g milk, accounting for approximately 80% of total energy intake. However, other foods were given and by 6 to 7 months of age about half the infants had received cereals and fruits and 20% had received dairy products, such as cow's or goat's milk.

The protection afforded by breast-feeding against diarrheal diseases may be less obvious in this area than in an area where children receive little or no breast milk. Nevertheless, 6- to 8-month-old infants who received 90% or more of their daily caloric intake from breast milk had less diarrhea than children of the same age who got a greater proportion of their intake from complementary foods (Table 1). Those infants getting more than 90% of their energy intake from breast milk were exclusively breast-fed. In the next 6 months of life, however, the more and less heavily breast-fed infants had similar rates of diarrhea. By this period of their life, nearly all infants had other foods introduced into their diet. The proportion of intake from other foods varied from child to child, but rarely contributed substantially to nutrient intake. On the other hand, the ingestion of even small quantities of heavily contaminated food could have increased the risk of diarrhea for these children.

TABLE 1. *Incidence of diarrhea in infants obtaining at least 90% or less than 90% of caloric intake from breast milk by age*

Age (months)	≥ 90% of Caloric intake from breast milk			< 90% of Caloric intake from breast milk		
	Months of observation	Episodes of diarrhea	Incidence per 100 months	Months of observation	Episodes of diarrhea	Incidence per 100 months
6–8	55	27	49	14	11	79
9–14	118	47	40	103	49	48
Total	173	74	43	117	60	51

TABLE 2. *Level of contamination with Escherichia coli in food consumed by weaning-aged children and relation to environmental temperature*

Food type; noontime indoor temperature (°F)	Number of specimens	Percentage of specimens by *E. coli* colony count per g or ml							Geometric mean colony count of specimens with *E. coli*
		0	10^0–10^1	10^2	10^3	10^4	10^5	10^6–10^7	
Rice									
< 75	85	79	9	5	4	2	1	—	4×10^2
75–84.9	113	72	4	4	11	3	4	3	4×10^3
≥85	130	48	4	13	15	11	5	4	6×10^3
Milk									
<75	25	64	12	24	—	—	—	—	1×10^2
75–84.9	28	57	14	7	11	4	—	7	7×10^2
≥85	20	25	—	—	20	10	40	5	6×10^4
Other									
< 75	14	64	14	14	—	7	—	—	5×10^2
75–84.9	24	58	8	8	—	17	8	—	4×10^3
≥85	31	23	3	3	10	32	23	6	3×10^4
Total	470	59	6	8	9	8	6	3	4×10^3

In the analysis of the bacteriological results, the presence of *Escherichia coli* in a food or water sample was regarded as evidence of fecal contamination (2). Of 470 food specimens, 70% were cooked rice, 16% were cow's or goat's milk, and 15% were other types of food, including special weaning foods made of rice or wheat flour and milk (Table 2). Forty-nine percent of milk specimens and 57% of the other types of food contained *E. coli*, compared with 37% of rice specimens. The frequency of contamination of foods with *E. coli* rose markedly with increasing environmental temperature.

The common practice of cooking foods early in the morning and storing them at ambient temperature for consumption later in the day appeared to encourage the growth of *E. coli*. On 20 occasions, milk was heated in the morning, some drunk immediately, and some later in the day; on 70% of these days the *E. coli* counts were higher, usually by 10-fold or more, after storage than they had been shortly after preparation. A similar relationship between storage time and *E. coli* counts was noted for other foods.

Of 475 drinking water specimens, 50% contained *E. coli*; however, the average number of *E. coli* in water was 10-fold lower than in food specimens.

We found that the proportion of foods containing *E. coli* was positively correlated with the children's annual incidence of diarrhea associated with enterotoxigenic *E. coli* (Fig. 1), but not with the incidence of rotavirus, *Shigella*, or other diarrheas. Drinking water contamination was not correlated with the incidence of any specific type of diarrhea.

In a two-year study at a treatment center in rural Bangladesh, *E. coli* diarrhea was found to have a marked seasonal distribution which was strikingly cor-

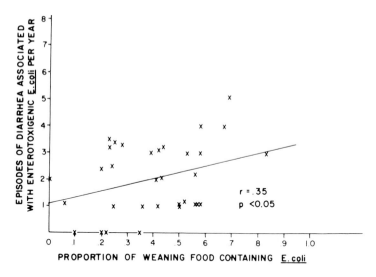

FIG. 1. Annual incidence of enterotoxigenic *E. coli* diarrhea for children 6 to 24 months old by proportion of weaning food specimens contaminated with *E. coli*.

related with the environmental temperature (Fig. 2). The seasonal variation in the level of contamination of foods is the most likely explanation for this seasonality of enterotoxigenic *E. coli* diarrhea.

Promotion and encouragement of breast-feeding is a very important strategy to reduce the incidence of diarrhea and its consequences—malnutrition and

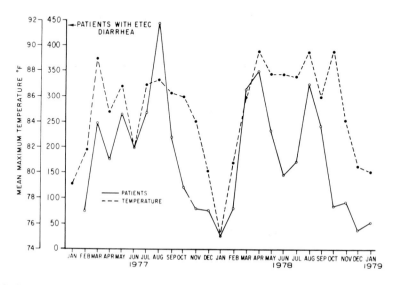

FIG. 2. Number of patients with enterotoxigenic *E. coli* diarrhea and ambient temperature.

death. At the same time, we must recognize the need of infants for adequate amounts and types of complementary foods. A recent WHO/UNICEF meeting recommended that "foods locally available in the home can be made suitable for weaning" (10). While we strongly endorse this concept, we must at the same time attempt to prevent fecal contamination of such foods. The studies presented here suggest that some diarrheas, particularly those due to the very frequent enterotoxigenic *E. coli*, could be prevented if these foods were prepared hygienically and eaten immediately, or stored safely until consumption. Practical and inexpensive approaches are needed to prevent the transmission of enteropathogens to infants in developing countries.

REFERENCES

1. Barrell, R. A. E., and Rowland, M. G. M. (1979): Infant foods as a potential source of diarrhoeal illness in rural West Africa. *Trans. R. Soc. Trop. Med. Hyg.*, 73:85–90.
2. Black, R. E., Brown, K. H., Becker, S., Alim, A. R. M. A., and Merson, M. H. (1982): Contamination of weaning foods and transmission of enterotoxigenic *Escherichia coli* diarrhoea in children in rural Bangladesh. *Trans. R. Soc. Trop. Med. Hyg.*, 76:259–264.
3. Brown, K. H., Black, R. E., Becker, S., Nahar, S., and Sawyer, J. (1982): Consumption of foods and nutrients by weanlings in rural Bangladesh. *Am. J. Clin. Nutr.*, 36:878–889.
4. Cunningham, A. S. (1979): Morbidity in breast-fed and artificially fed infants. II. *J. Pediatr.*, 95:685–689.
5. Mata, L. J. (1975): Malnutrition-infection interactions in the tropics. *Am. J. Trop. Med. Hyg.*, 24:564–574.
6. Mata, L., Jiménez, P., Allen, M. A., Vargas, W., García, M. E., Urrutia, J. J., and Wyatt, R. G. (1981): Diarrhea and malnutrition: breastfeeding intervention in a transitional population. In: *Acute Enteric Infections in Children. New Prospects for Treatment and Prevention*, pp. 233–259. Elsevier/North-Holland, Amsterdam.
7. Scrimshaw, N. S., Taylor, C. E., and Gordon, J. E. (1968): *Interactions of Nutrition and Infection*. WHO Monograph, Ser. No. 57.
8. Watkinson, M. (1981): Delayed onset of weaning diarrhoea associated with high breast milk intake. *Trans. R. Soc. Trop. Med. Hyg.*, 75:432–435.
9. Welsh, J. K., and May, J. T. (1979): Anti-infective properties of breast milk. *J. Pediatr.*, 94:1–9.
10. WHO/UNICEF Meeting (1979): *Lancet*, ii:841–843.

Acute Diarrhea: Its Nutritional Consequences in Children, edited by J. A. Bellanti.
Nestlé, Vevey/Raven Press, New York © 1983.

EPIDEMIOLOGY OF ACUTE DIARRHEA IN CHILDHOOD

Discussion

Dr. Suskind: In the last community you referred to, what were the specific measures you took to achieve such a dramatic change?

Dr. Mata: This is a long-term study of a large, typical rural population with a very active rural health program and a good water supply. In addition, we have initiated an intervention program in the hospital where most of the women deliver their babies. The custom in that hospital was to separate the infant from the mother. We did change that. We put the mother and infant together. We tried to promote breast-feeding by placing a psychologist in the hospital to work with the mothers and teach them how to breast-feed. We have been very successful with this program of inducing breast-feeding to the extent that more than 85% of the infants are breast-fed exclusively for at least 2 months. Further, a rural health program of immunization assures that every child is vaccinated. After 4 years of field work, 1,700 infants have been vaccinated against the usual diseases of childhood—measles, whooping cough, and so forth, and we have not had any deaths due to diarrhea either in 3 years.

Dr. Klish: I would like to make a comment about the incidence figures with regard to diarrhea. We just have completed a study in Rochester on the incidence of diarrhea in children; this was done in an out-patient setting rather than an in-patient setting. To my knowledge most of the incidence figures that we have, at least in the United States, are related to those severe forms of diarrhea that are presented to the hospitals or to clinics that deal with severe diarrhea. In this study we enrolled 500 patients, of whom about 250 were infected with rotavirus. Out of the 500 patients, only one required rehydration above and behind a telephone call to the doctor's office. So it may be that in the United States there is a much higher incidence of diarrhea than previously thought, but the difference is that the disease here is very mild as compared with some other countries.

Dr. Bellanti: What was the age spectrum of those children?

Dr. Klish: The data have not yet been completely analyzed, but I would expect that about two-thirds of the infants were less than 1 year of age.

Dr. Mata: We have the impression in Costa Rica that the children of wealthy families who go to private pediatricians also have a very high incidence of diarrhea, but it's mild. I think the explanation is that in clean environments those children get low infectious doses, and there is a high correlation between severity and infectious dose.

Dr. Klish: I believe you are correct in what you said. In our study, we are going to be able to quantitate the rotavirus load and it appears that those children who are more significantly ill definitely have a higher colony count in their colon. I do not know if this relates to the dose of infective organism.

Dr. Santosham: I wanted to respond to Dr. Suskind's question about what can be done in this country about reduction of mortality. There is an example in this country of dramatic reduction in the mortality rate in a reservation of Apaches in Arizona. In 1973, the mortality rate was anywhere from 80 to 100 per thousand. Now they are below the national average. What happened between then and now is as follows: Sanitation was introduced. Besides sanitation, an oral rehydration program was introduced. Mothers were taught to bring children into the hospital quickly for diarrhea. Another aspect of the program is the maternal and child health program which is called the Pride of the Apaches. The midwives visit the homes, educate the parents, and conduct an active program of immunization.

The results of a study of children infected with rotavirus as neonates are as follows. We identified 2 groups of children, one of whom excreted rotavirus in the first 2 weeks of life and another who showed no evidence of rotavirus excretion during the first 2 weeks. We followed up these children for 3 years with 3-monthly sera. The children who excreted rotavirus during the first 2 weeks experienced another episode of rotavirus during the first 3 years. Most of those children were asymptomatic, and the ones who did have symptoms had relatively mild ones. The infants who were negative during the first 2 weeks after birth and who became infected with rotavirus for the first time after the neonatal period had a symptomatic infection with a tendency toward severity, and, in fact, three of those children required hospital admission.

Acute Diarrhea: Its Nutritional Consequences
in Children, edited by J. A. Bellanti.
Nestlé, Vevey/Raven Press, New York © 1983.

ETIOLOGIC AGENTS OF ACUTE DIARRHEA

In Vitro Cultivation of Human Rotavirus in MA104 Cells

Tasuke Konno, Toyoko Kutsuzawa, and Hiroshi Suzuki

Department of Pediatrics, Tohoku University School of Medicine, Sendai 980, Japan

Recently, viruses or virus-like particles have been detected by electron microscopic examination in stools from patients with acute diarrhea; they are considered the causative agents of acute diarrhea (3). Among them, the human rotavirus has been recognized as a most important pathogen of acute diarrhea in infants and young children in many parts of the world. However, these viruses associated with acute diarrhea have been identified mainly on the basis of their morphological and immunological features. Although a great deal of effort has been directed to adaptation of these viruses to continued propagation in cell cultures, only several animal viruses, including rotavirus strains, have been adapted to grow efficiently to high titer in cell culture (13). The difficulties in propagating human enteric viruses, particularly rotavirus in conventional cell culture systems, have hampered rapid progress in virological, serological, and epidemiological studies on viral diarrheal diseases.

In 1980, the Wa strain, human rotavirus type 2, was first adapted to grow efficiently in primary, green monkey, kidney cell cultures after passages in newborn gnotobiotic piglets (12). Most recently, successful *in vitro* cultivation systems for human rotavirus, without any passages in animals, were reported by Sato et al. (10) and subsequently confirmed by Urasawa et al. (11). On the basis of these results, it was suggested that most human rotaviruses could be cultivated in cell cultures. In view of such successful cultivation, we attempted to cultivate in cell cultures human rotaviruses that had been serotyped either subgroup 1 or subgroup 2 by immune adherence hemagglutination (IAHA) or enzyme-linked immunosorbent assay (ELISA) (5), and succeeded in isolating two tissue culture-adapted strains distinguishable from each other by IAHA (8). This chapter describes the methods for cultivating these two isolates in MA104 cell cultures.

MATERIALS AND METHODS

The fecal specimens for this study were obtained from infants with acute diarrhea and stored at −80°C. Rotavirus particles in these specimens had been previously detected by electron microscopy (EM).

31

The ribonucleic acid (RNA) profiles of these rotavirus strains were analyzed by a polyacrylamide gel electrophoresis. For electrophoresis, the rotaviruses were purified by the method previously reported (7). The purified viruses were deproteinized with phenol, and the RNA was precipitated with ethanol. The pelleted RNA was dissolved in Laemmli's sample buffer (9). After electrophoresis, the gels were stained with ethidium bromide solution. As shown in Table 1, the rotavirus of specimen 80SR004 was observed to have an RNA pattern with slow-moving segments 10 and 11 and was designated S type. The virus of 80SP001 exhibited an RNA pattern with fast-moving segments 10 and 11 and was designated L type. The RNA patterns, S and L type, correspond as far as segments 10 and 11 are concerned to 2s and 2l, respectively, as described by Espejo et al. (2).

Subgroup specificities were examined by ELISA and/or IAHA in collaboration with A. Z. Kapikian (National Institutes of Health, Bethesda, Maryland) (7), revealing that the rotavirus strain with an RNA pattern of S type belonged to subgroup 1 and the L type to subgroup 2.

For virus isolation in cell culture, an established cell line (MA104) derived from the kidney of an embryonal, rhesus monkey was used. Growth medium for MA104 cell culture was Eagle's minimum essential medium (MEM), supplemented with 10% fetal calf serum (FCS) and antibiotics (100 units penicillin and 100 μg streptomycin). Maintenance medium was MEM containing 0.5 μg/ml trypsin (Sigma IX), antibiotics, and no serum. All cultures were incubated at 37°C. The cultures for virus isolation were incubated in a roller drum.

For inoculation, 10% homogenous suspensions of fecal specimens were made in MEM and centrifuged successively at 3,000 rpm and 10,000 rpm. The clarified supernatant was mixed with an equal amount of 20 μg/ml trypsin and incubated at 37°C for 20 min. Before inoculation, the trypsin-treated fecal specimens were diluted 1:20 with MEM.

To ascertain virus growth in cell culture, every culture medium was examined by EM after staining with 1% uranyl acetate solution.

RESULTS

Isolation and Propagation of Rotaviruses in Cell Cultures

Confluent monolayer cultures of MA104 cells prepared in 10 × 110 mm culture tubes were washed with maintenance medium and then inoculated with 0.2 ml of the 1:20 diluted trypsin-treated fecal specimens. After 1 hr adsorption at 37°C, cell cultures were washed with MEM without serum, suspended in the maintenance medium containing trypsin, and then incubated in a roller drum. The media were changed every other day and checked by EM for the presence of virus particles. On the 11th day after the initial inoculation, the culture tubes were frozen and thawed three times, and centrifuged at 3,000 rpm. The supernatants of the culture lysates were treated with

TABLE 1. *Source of isolates*

Patient	Sex	Onset of diarrhea	Collection of stool	EM	RNA	Subgroup
Takiguchi (80SR004)	F	Jan. 12, 1980	Jan. 16, 1980	+++	S[a]	1
Nagatsuka (80SP001)	M	Feb. 1, 1980	Feb. 6, 1980	++	L[a]	2

[a] S: slow-moving segments 10 and 11; L: fast-moving segments 10 and 11.

trypsin and then inoculated into fresh confluent cell monolayer cultures for the second passage.

On the second passage, the culture tubes were frozen on day 6 after inoculation and, following trypsin treatment, the culture fluids were inoculated onto fresh MA104 cell monolayers in tubes. On subsequent passages, the culture fluid for the next passage was obtained 2 or 3 days after inoculation.

Cytopathic effects were observed 10 days postinfection during the primary passage in one out of four culture tubes inoculated with stool specimens 80SR004 (Takiguchi), and 8 days postinfection in two out of four tubes, and 9 days in three out of four tubes with specimens 80SP001 (Nagatsuka). The cultivated rotavirus strain derived from 80SR004 was named KUN and that from 80SP001 was named MO. On the second passage, cytopathic effects were noticed at day 4 in one, day 5 in two, and day 6 in three out of four culture tubes with KUN; and at day 4 in two, day 5 in three, and day 6 in four out of four tubes with MO. However, distinct cytopathic effects were observed on the sixth passage with KUN, and the third passage with MO (Table 2). Thereafter, cytopathic effects were recognized 48 to 72 hr after infection. The cytopathic effects consisted of obscure cell boundary, cell fusion, cell rounding, cell detaching, and lytic foci.

Rotavirus particles in the culture media were detected by EM on the second and subsequent passages, and the number of viruses detected increased when passages progressed. Most of the virus particles found in the culture media had

TABLE 2. *Occurrence of CPE and detection by EM of rotavirus particles in MA104 cells*

Strain		Passage in MA104 cells				
	1st	2nd	3rd	4th	5th	6th
KUN CPE	±	+	+	+	+	+++
EM	−	+	++	++−+++	++−+++	+++
MO CPE	±	+	++++	+++	+++	+++
EM	−	+	++−+++	+++	+++	+++

a characteristic appearance of rotavirus with a double capsid. Empty particles or virus lacking an outer capsid were infrequently observed.

The infectious titer of the culture fluids was $10^7 TCID_{50}/ml$ in KUN on the eighth passage, and $10^{7.5} TCID_{50}/ml$ in MO on the seventh passage in a roller tube culture.

RNA Patterns of Human Rotavirus Isolates KUN and MO

To establish the identity of the tissue culture-adapted rotavirus strains, viral RNA was examined by a polyacrylamide gel electrophoresis. In our laboratory, animal rotaviruses had never been used for investigation, but Wa strain cultivable human rotavirus had been grown and investigated. Considering the ease with which cultures could be contaminated, RNA profiles of the strains KUN and MO were compared not only with those of their original fecal viruses, but also with the RNA profile of the Wa strain that had been thoroughly investigated. Rotaviruses subjected to RNA analysis were obtained in confluent cell monolayers in roller bottles infected with the sixth passage KUN and fifth passage MO. The electrophoretic RNA patterns of the isolated rotavirus strains KUN and MO were found to be identical to those of their respective original viruses (Table 3). They were different in electrophoretic RNA pattern from the Wa strain. The isolate KUN was S type and MO was L type, as far as mobility of RNA segments 10 and 11 was concerned.

Antigenic Specificities of the Tissue Culture-Adapted
Rotavirus KUN and MO

Subgroup specificity of the isolates grown in MA104 cell cultures was examined by IAHA in collaboration with A. Z. Kapikian, and compared with the original viruses. The KUN virus was identified as subgroup 1, and the MO virus as subgroup 2; these were the same subgroups as the rotaviruses present in the stools of the patients Takiguchi and Nagatsuka (Table 3).

Growth in Stationary Cultures of Isolates KUN and MO

Attempts to adapt the isolates to stationary cultures first succeeded on the 11th passage with KUN strain and on the eighth passage with MO strain.

TABLE 3. *Comparison of RNA patterns and subgroup specificities of isolated human rotavirus by tissue culture and their origins*

	Fecal 80SR004 (Takiguchi)	Cultivated KUN	Fecal 80SP001 (Nagatsuka)	Cultivated MO
RNA[a]	S	S	L	L
IAHA Subgroup	1	1	2	2

[a] Identical in mobility of all RNA segments between S types, and between L types.

However, their infectious titer in stationary culture was much lower than that in roller tube culture. The infectious titer of the first stationary cultures was $10^{2.5}$TCID$_{50}$/ml with both KUN and MO strains. In addition, cytopathic changes were not as distinct as in roller cultures.

DISCUSSION

Initial Isolation of the Virus

The present study confirmed the *in vitro* cultivation method of human rotaviruses, which had been reported previously by Sato et al. and Urasawa et al. in Japan (10,11). In this experiment, however, the incubation period was prolonged until cytopathic changes appeared on the first and second passage, while in previous reports passages had been made at intervals of 3 days or 3 to 5 days (10,11). Urasawa et al. concentrated the culture fluid by centrifugation before inoculation on the second and third passages (11). The adaptation procedure adopted by different authors is therefore somewhat difficult, but the fact remains that successful *in vitro* cultivations have been made independently in three laboratories. This could suggest that most rotavirus strains could be adapted to grow efficiently and undergo serial passages with a growth yield sufficient to permit characterization of the virus.

Wa strain is the first cell culture of an adapted human rotavirus. However, serial passage of the Wa strain in cell culture was achieved only with the 11th passage material from newborn gnotobiotic piglets (12).

Sato et al. (10), having been successful in the primary isolation of human rotavirus in cell culture, emphasized the importance of using MA104 cells, pretreating the virus with trypsin, and adding trypsin in the maintenance medium. In addition, they used a roller tube culture that was supposed to produce more pronounced cytopathic effect with bovine rotavirus than a stationary culture (6).

Appearance of Cytopathic Effects

Although the early reports of the cytopathic effect with bovine rotavirus included a description of "flagging," where cells are partially detached from the surface and wave in the medium, as being characteristic and even diagnostic for rotavirus-infected monolayers (3), this has not been generally accepted. Cytopathic effect was also described to take the form of nondescript granular degeneration of the cell monolayer (13). In this study, cytopathic effects with KUN and MO strains included obscure cell borders, cell fusion, cell rounding, cell piling-up, cell-detaching from the surface of the tubes, and lytic foci. Thus, the appearance of cytopathic effects with the virus strains was easily recognized in the cell culture, but its true nature was not well characterized.

Because of the slow and inapparent development of cytopathic effects, the increase of the number of virus particles detected by EM in culture media provided a good aid to determine the day of virus harvest in the culture.

Although immunofluorescent staining is known to be useful for detecting virus growth in cell cultures (10,11), it was not performed in this study.

Use of Trypsin

The experience with isolates of animal rotavirus as well as of Wa strain has suggested that the use of trypsin is essential in the cultivation (13). In the case of human rotavirus strains adapted to grow in cell cultures by Japanese investigators, the inoculum was treated with trypsin and the latter was also added to the maintenance medium (10,11). In this study, the concentration of trypsin used was 10 μg/ml for virus treatment prior to inoculation and 0.5 μg/ml for maintenance medium; MA104 cells could tolerate this concentration. While the mechanism of action has not been elucidated, trypsin is presumed to exert an effect on the virus itself by cleaving surface polypeptide(s) and to act on progeny viruses produced in the early replication cycles (13).

Virus Plaquing

We attempted to propagate the roller culture-adapted rotavirus strains, KUN and MO, in a stationary cell culture that would offer the advantage of characterizing the virus. In the case of the isolate KUN, the virus was adapted to a stationary culture in MA104 cells on passage 11, and in the MO strain on passage 7. Plaque formation with these viruses is now in progress. The Wa strain and the virus strains isolated by Urasawa et al. are adapted to produce plaques in MA104 monolayer culture, which is also enhanced by the addition of trypsin in agar overlays (11,12). Efforts for plaquing should be continued to facilitate serological characterization as well as genetic manipulation of the virus.

Electrophoretypes and Serotypes

The electrophoretic migration patterns of tissue culture-adapted human rotavirus KUN and MO were identical to those of original fecal viruses, confirming the isolates to be human rotaviruses.

Although antigenic properties of rotavirus have not been throughly understood, the existence of more than two serotypes has been evidenced by a variety of methods including complement fixation, ELISA, IAHA, and neutralization (1,5,14). Recently, evidence of the dissociation of neutralization and IAHA antigenic specificities has been recognized in studies of human and bovine rotavirus reassortants (5). In addition, the existence of a correlation between the RNA patterns of human rotaviruses and their antigenic subgroup specificities has been demonstrated (4). The KUN and MO strains isolated in this study were identified by IAHA as subgroups 1 and 2, respectively, belonging to the same subgroups as the rotaviruses present in the stools. Correlation between the subgroup specificity and RNA patterns of the isolates KUN and MO was shown to be similar to that of the original stool rotaviruses.

In view of these results, neither KUN nor MO grown in MA104 cells appear to be contaminants of tissue culture-adapted human rotavirus, Wa strain, or animal rotaviruses.

It is of interest to note that KUN strain, belonging to subgroup 1, seemed reluctant to grow in cell culture, especially on early passages, compared with MO strain, subgroup 2. Although still unproven, this may be caused by antigenic differences of human rotaviruses.

The successful cultivation of two human rotavirus KUN and MO strains with different antigenic properties in subgroup specificity correlated with electrophoretic RNA pattern might facilitate a detailed study of the viruses. The methods of culture for human rotavirus should be useful for other viruses causing acute diarrhea.

ACKNOWLEDGEMENT

The authors are indebted to Dr. A. Z. Kapikian of National Institutes of Health, USA, for his generous help with serological examinations of rotavirus strains.

REFERENCES

1. Beards, G. M., Pilforld, J. N., Thouless, M. E., and Flewett, T. H. (1980): Rotavirus serotypes by serum neutralization. *J. Med. Virol.*, 5:231–237.
2. Espejo, R. T., Calderon, E., Gonzalez, N., Salomon, A., Mortuscelli, M., and Romero, P. (1979): Presence of two distinct types of rotavirus in infants and young children hospitalized with acute gastroenteritis in Mexico City, 1977. *J. Infect. Dis.*, 139:474–477.
3. Holmes, I. H. (1979): Viral gastroenteritis. *Prog. Med. Virol.*, 25:1–36.
4. Kalica, A. R., Greenberg, H. B., Espejo, R. T., Flores, J., Wyatt, R. G., Kapikian, A. Z., and Chanock, R. M. (1981): Distinctive ribonucleic acid patterns of human rotavirus subgroups 1 and 2. *Infect. Immun.*, 33:958–961.
5. Kapikian, A. Z., Cline, W. L., Greenberg, H. B., Wyatt, R. G., Kalica, A. R., Banks, C. E., James, H. D., Jr., Flores, J., and Chanock, R. M. (1981): Antigenic characterization of human and animal rotaviruses by immune adherence hemagglutination assay (IAHA): Evidence for distinctness of IAHA and neutralization antigens. *Infect. Immun.*, 33:415–425.
6. Kurogi, H., Inaba, Y., Takahashi, E., Sato, K., Goto, Y., and Omori, T. (1976): Cytopathic effect of Nebraska calf diarrhea virus (Lincoln strain) on secondary bovine kidney cell monolayer. *Natl. Inst. Anim. Health Q. Tokyo*, 16:133–136.
7. Kutsuzawa, T., Konno, T., Suzuki, H., Ebina, T., and Ishida, N. (1982): Two distinct electrophoretic migration patterns of RNA segments of human rotavirus prevalent in Japan in relation to their serotypes. *Microbiol. Immunol.*, 26:271–273.
8. Kutsuzawa, T., Konno, T., Suzuki, H., Kapikian, A. Z., Ebina, T., and Ishida, N. (1982): Isolation of human rotavirus subgroup 1 and 2 in cell culture. *J. Clin. Microbiol.*, 16:727–730.
9. Laemmli, U. K. (1970): Cleavage of structural proteins during the assembly of the head of bacteriophage T$_4$. *Nature*, 227:680–685.
10. Sato, K., Inaba, Y., Shinozuka, T., Fujii, R., and Matsumoto, M. (1981): Isolation of human rotavirus in cell cultures. *Arch. Virol.*, 69:155–160.
11. Urasawa, T., Urasawa, S., and Taniguchi, K. (1981): Sequential passages of human rotavirus in MA-104 cells. *Microbiol. Immunol.*, 25:1025–1035.
12. Wyatt, R. G., James, W. D., Bohl, E. H., Theil, K. W., Saif, L. J., Kalica, A. R., Greenberg, H. B., Kapikian, A. Z., and Chanock, R. M. (1980): Human rotavirus type 2: cultivation *in vitro*. *Science*, 207:189–191.
13. Wyatt, R. G., and James, N. D. (1981): Methods of virus culture *in vivo* and *in vitro*. In: *Virus Infection of the Gastrointestinal Tract*, edited by D. A. Tyrrel and A. Z. Kapikian. Marcel Dekker, New York.
14. Zissis, G., and Lambert, J. P. (1978): Different serotypes of human rotavirus. *Lancet*, 1:38–39.

Acute Diarrhea: Its Nutritional Consequences in Children, edited by J. A. Bellanti.
Nestlé, Vevey/Raven Press, New York © 1983.

ETIOLOGIC AGENTS OF ACUTE DIARRHEA

Adenoviruses as Etiologic Agents of Acute Gastroenteritis

Robert H. Yolken

Division of Infectious Diseases, Johns Hopkins University School of Medicine, Baltimore, Maryland 21205

The recent elucidation of etiologic agents of infantile diarrhea has markedly improved our understanding of the pathophysiology and epidemiology of acute nonbacterial gastroenteritis. In addition, the study of these agents has led to the formulation of potential strategies for the prevention and treatment of these infections. The agent of nonbacterial gastroenteritis in children which has received the most attention is human rotavirus. This agent is responsible for a large percentage of the serious cases of diarrhea which occur in children living in both developed and developing countries (3,8). However, in spite of the importance of this agent, it is clear that there are numerous episodes of serious diarrheal disease which cannot be explained by infection with rotavirus or with known bacterial agents.

Studies in our population have indicated that some of these cases of gastroenteritis are caused by adenoviruses. These viruses are icosahedral, nonlipid-containing DNA viruses, which are capable of replicating in multiple body sites, including the respiratory and gastrointestinal tracts (7). To study the role of adenoviruses in acute diarrhea, we devised enzyme immunoassays for the measurement of adenoviral antigens in stool specimens. We utilized reagents directed at hexon antigen to detect common adenoviral antigen in the stool specimens (5). We then further characterized the adenovirus by the use of reagents specifically directed at adenoviruses implicated in diarrheal disease. These adenoviruses, which have been tentatively designated adenovirus type 38 and type 39, can be distinguished from other adenoviruses by their antigenic makeup and DNA restriction patterns (6). In addition, these adenoviruses are not cultivable in human, embryonic, kidney cells and other cell lines utilized to grow adenoviruses obtained from the respiratory tract (2). These adenoviruses are, thus, similar to other viruses causing diarrhea such as rotavirus and Norwalk virus, which are difficult to cultivate in *in vitro* systems (1).

We utilized these immunoassay systems to examine the role of adenoviruses as causes of infantile gastroenteritis in our population. We concentrated on the fall months, since previous studies in our population have documented

TABLE 1. Clinical characteristics of infants with diarrhea associated with enteric-type adenovirus and other agents

Agent identified	No. of patients	Mean age (months)	Mean (range) duration of diarrhea (days)	Mean maximum no. stools/day	No. (%) with signs or symptoms				
					Temperature (> 38.5°C)	Vomiting	Conjunctivitis	Respiratory[a]	Pneumonia[b]
Enteric-type adenovirus	14	8.2	8.0[c] (2–16)	8.5	13 (93)[c]	11 (79)[c]	3 (21)	13 (93)[c]	6 (43)[c]
Other adenovirus	2	8.6	5.0 (4–6)	7.5	1 (50)	0	0	1 (50)	0
Salmonella enteriditis	2	9.0	6.0 (5–7)	8.5	1 (50)	0	0	1 (50)	0
No agent identified	9	8.3	3.6 (2–8)	8.1	4 (44)	3 (33)	0	3 (33)	0

[a] Respiratory symptoms consisted of wheezing, coryza, cough, or rhinorrhea.
[b] Definite infiltrate noted by pulmonary radiography.
[c] $p < 0.05$ by Fischer's exact test (2-tailed) or t-test (2-tailed) when compared to all diarrhea other than that caused by enteric-type adenovirus.

that this is a period in which a large number of cases of acute gastroenteritis occur which could not be associated with known infectious agents. Our studies indicated that adenoviruses could be identified in the stools of a large number of children who were inpatients in our institution during the fall months. Virtually all of the children infected with enteric types of adenovirus had serious diarrhea. In addition, most of the children had respiratory symptoms, and half of the children had severe pneumonia as evidenced by infiltrates and chest X-rays (Table 1). Also, a serological response to enteric adenovirus was found in children from whom appropriate sera were available. These findings suggest that adenoviruses are important causes of diarrheal disease in our population at certain times of the year. Continued surveillance has revealed that adenoviruses are associated with approximately 15% of the cases of serious diarrhea in our population. In periods when rotavirus is not prevalent, adenoviruses can be found in more than 40% of the cases of serious diarrhea. Preliminary studies of the acquisition of antibody to enteric type adenovirus indicate that infection is widespread with half of our children having such antibody by 3 years of age. Infection appears to be even more widespread in other populations with over 98% of children living in some areas showing serological evidence of infections by 3 years of age.

Another population with high rate of adenovirus gastroenteritis are patients who are immunocompromised. A prospective study of patients undergoing bone marrow transplantation revealed 11 with adenovirus infection. Virtually all of these patients had severe diarrhea and most had severe respiratory disease (Table 2). In addition, many of these patients died within 2 weeks of their

TABLE 2. *Relation of the enteric pathogens to clinical symptoms in immunocompromised patients*

Pathogen	No. patients	No. with indicated symptoms				
		Vomiting	Diarrhea	Abdominal cramps	Respiratory illness	Death
Rotavirus	8	8	4	7	6	5
Adenovirus[a]	9	8	5	5	4	4
Coxsackie virus[a]	2	1	2	1	1	2
Rotavirus and adenovirus[c]	1	1	0	0	0	0
Coxsackie and adenovirus[ab]	2	1	2	2	2	2
Any viral pathogen	22	19	13[e]	15[e]	13[d]	13[e]
C. difficile only	9	6	5[d]	4	3	4
Any pathogen	31	25	18[e]	19[e]	16[d]	17[d]
No virus or toxin	47	31	6	6	9	6

[a] Includes one patient coinfected with *C. difficile* toxin within 6 weeks of the viral infection.
[b] Both patients were simultaneously infected with coxsackie virus and adenovirus.
[c] The onset of the rotavirus and adenovirus infections was separated by a 4-week interval. The vomiting occurred within 5 days of the rotavirus infection.
[d] $p < 0.05$ compared with no virus or toxin. Statistical analyses were not performed for the individual viruses.
[e] $p < 0.001$ compared with no virus or toxin.

adenovirus infection. These findings highlight the severe nature of adenovirus gastroenteritis in children who become immunoincompetent during the course of cancer chemotherapy. These findings also suggest that the role of adenovirus in immunodeficiencies associated with malnutrition and metabolic diseases should be further investigated.

Further studies should be directed at elucidating the epidemiology and pathophysiology of adenovirus gastroenteritis. The availability of specific antisera to detect adenovirus types associated with diarrhea should make this task more feasible. In addition, further studies should be directed at measuring adenoviruses in environmental sources to determine better the mode of transmission of enteric adenovirus infections. The high rate of respiratory disease associated with adenovirus gastroenteritis also suggests that the effect of respiratory disease in the efficacy of oral hydration programs needs to be investigated. Finally, the availability of vaccines for the prevention of respiratory adenoviruses (4) suggests that vaccines for enteric type adenoviruses could be developed. The elimination of adenovirus gastroenteritis might represent a major step in the decrease of the morbidity and mortality associated with viral gastroenteritis.

REFERENCES

1. Greenberg, H. B., Wyatt, R. G., Kalica, A. R., Yolken, R. H., Black, R., Kapikian, A. Z., and Chanock, R. M. (1981): New insights in viral gastroenteritis. *Perspect. Virol.*, XI:163–187.
2. Johanssan, M. E., Unhou, I., Kidd, A. H., et al. (1980): Direct identification of enteric adenovirus, a candidate new serotype associated with infantile gastroenteritis. *J. Clin. Microbiol.*, 12:95.
3. Kapikian, A. Z., Kim, H. W., Wyatt, R. C., Cline, W. L., Arrobio, J. O., Brandt, C. D., Rodrigues, W. J., Sack, D. A., Chanock, R. M., and Parrott, R. H. (1976): Human reovirus like agent as the major pathogen associated with "winter" gastroenteritis in hospitalized infants and young children. *N. Engl. J. Med.*, 294:965.
4. Kasel, J. A., Alford, R. H., Lehrich, J. R. et al. (1966): Adenovirus soluble antigens for human immunization. *Am. Rev. Resp. Dis.*, 94:170–174.
5. Sarkkinen, H. K., Tuokko, H. and Halonen, P. E. (1980): Comparison of enzyme immunoassay and radioimmunoassay for detection of human rotaviruses and adenoviruses from stool specimens. *J. Virol. Methods*, 1:331–341.
6. Takiff, H. E., Straus, S. E., and Garen, C. E. (1981): Propagation and *in vitro* studies of previously non-cultivatable enteral adenoviruses in 293 cells. *Lancet*, 7:832.
7. Wadell, G., Hammarskjuld, M. L., Winberg, G., et al. (1980): Genetic variability of adenoviruses, *Ann. NY Acad. Sci.*, 354:16.
8. Wyatt, R. G., Yolken, G. H., Urrutia, J. J. et al. (1979): Diarrhea associated with rotavirus in rural Guatemala: A longitudinal study of 24 infants and young children. *Am. J. Trop. Med. Hyg.*, 28:325.

Acute Diarrhea: Its Nutritional Consequences in Children, edited by J. A. Bellanti.
Nestlé, Vevey/Raven Press, New York © 1983.

Etiologic Agents of Acute Diarrhea

Selected Aspects of Pathogenesis of Human and Murine Rotavirus Infections

*†‡Marie Riepenhoff-Talty, §Hiroshi Suzuki, and *†‡Pearay L. Ogra

*Departments of *Pediatrics and †Microbiology, State University of New York at Buffalo, Buffalo, New York 14214; ‡School of Medicine and Division of Infectious Diseases and Virology, Children's Hospital, Buffalo, New York 14222; and §University of Nagasaki, Nagasaki, Japan*

Following the important discovery by Bishop and her colleagues in 1973 (1) that reovirus-like particles in duodenal biopsies of children with diarrhea had an etiologic relationship to their enteritis, the study of rotaviruses and the disease they produce has been intense. While the inability to cultivate human rotavirus *in vitro* retarded some studies, the availability of animal models in which species-specific rotaviruses produced nearly an identical disease were an obvious advantage (2,3,4,9). One prominent similarity between rotavirus-induced enteritis in humans and other mammals was the age restriction of serious disease to the young. In human infants the peak age appears to be 8 to 16 months; in mice it is 5 to 10 days. This age restriction is not well understood.

The present studies had a twofold purpose related to the pathogenesis of the infection. In humans and in mice, the relationship of the length of diarrhea was compared with virus replication either by monitoring virus shedding or by the detection of rotavirus antigen-positive cells. Second, in the mouse model, we studied the virus-enterocyte interaction. We isolated enterocytes from both suckling and adult, infected and uninfected mice, in an effort to explore the age dependence of the infection.

MATERIALS AND METHODS

Human Study Population

Forty infants hospitalized with rotavirus-induced gastroenteritis from whom we could obtain serial fecal samples were included in these studies. The patient population was selected at random and consisted of a slightly higher number of males than females.

Mouse Study Population

Swiss mice, randomly bred, ranging in age from 2 days to 6 months, were obtained commercially from the West Seneca Breeding Laboratory, West Seneca, New York. All animals were maintained in strict isolation facilities after virus inoculation. Groups of mice were inoculated with mouse rotavirus (MRV) according to the following schedule. Mice, 2 to 8 days of age, were administered approximately 0.1 ml of the virus intraorally by instillation. Mice, 9 to 24 days of age and over 25 days of age, were inoculated with about 0.1 ml and 0.2 ml, respectively, of the virus administered via nasogastric instillation. The animals in each age group were sacrificed 24 hr after the inoculation of the virus, and intestinal epithelial cells were prepared from segments of proximal small intestines, and noninfected age-matched controls inoculated with physiologic saline were included for each infected group and studied in an identical manner.

Mouse Rotavirus

MRV (EDIM 5099) was kindly supplied by Dr. Richard Wyatt (National Institutes of Health, Bethesda, Maryland). The virus pools were prepared from the homogenate of small intestine of 7- to 10-day-old suckling mice infected with MRV stock. The MRV-infected intestinal homogenates were clarified by centrifugation at 7,000 rpm to remove heavy cellular debris. The supernatant fluid was further concentrated and purified by ultracentrifugation and sucrose gradient.

Electron Microscopy

A small amount of sample, mixed with 2% ammonium acetate, was placed on a carbon-formvar coated copper mesh grid (Ernest Fullum Co., Schenectady, New York). After removal of excess sample with filter paper, a drop of 1% phosphotungstate (PTA), pH 7.2, was added to the grid. After approximately 1 min, the excess PTA was removed and the grid was placed 2 inches from an ultraviolet light for 3 to 5 min to inactivate viral infectivity. Following this procedure, the grid was examined for rotavirus particles with the aid of an electron microscope (JEOL, Tokyo, Japan).

Isolation of Enterocytes

Epithelial cells were dissociated from the duodenum and jejunum of uninfected or infected mice using a modification of the procedure described by Weiser (8). In brief, a 6- to 8-cm segment of the proximal small intestine was removed. The segment was dissected free of fat and connective tissue and cut open longitudinally. The tissue was washed in a balanced buffered saline solution containing 0.2% bovine serum albumin and agitated gently in a solution containing 0.5 mM ethyldiaminetetraacetate (EDTA). The resulting dissociated cells were washed three times and further testing was carried out.

Coating of Red Blood Cells with MRV

MRV was attached to sheep red blood cells (SRBC) by an adaptation of the technique of Poston (6) using chromium chloride. In brief, SRBC were suspended in piperazine buffer (pH 6.5) and incubated at room temperature with 0.1 ml of purified MRV in the presence of 2.25 M chromium chloride for 4 min.

RBC-MRV-Enterocyte Rosetting

Washed, isolated intestinal enterocytes obtained from uninfected animals of different age groups were mixed with an equal volume (0.1 ml) of MRV-coated RBC. The mixtures were centrifuged at 700 rpm for 5 min and the pellet of enterocytes and MRV-coated RBC was separated and incubated at 4°C for 30 min. The preparation was examined on a hemacytometer with a light microscope for the presence of RBC rosettes with enterocytes. At least 2,000 enterocytes were examined in each preparation. Binding of three or more RBC to an enterocyte was considered as an enterocyte-RBC rosette (Fig. 1).

Immunofluorescence for MRV in Enterocytes

The enterocytes obtained from infected mice were tested for the presence of MRV by employing direct immunofluorescence. Air-dried smears of

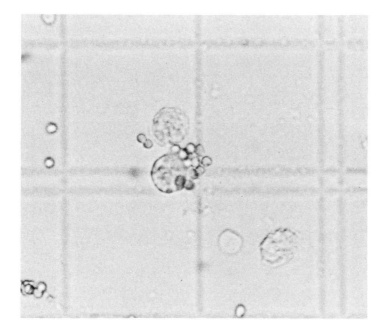

FIG. 1. Micrograph of an enterocyte-SRBC^{MRV} rosette (×600).

washed, dispersed, intestinal enterocytes were made on glass slides, fixed in acetone at 4°C for 10 min, and stained with a 1:20 dilution of fluorescin isothiocyanate (FITC)-conjugated antirotavirus serum for 45 min at 37°C. The cells were washed three times in phosphate-buffered saline (PBS) and read on a microscope equipped with a mercury vapor bulb (Leitz, Ortholux, Wetzlar, Germany).

Enzyme Immunoassay Technique

The "sandwich" enzyme-linked immunoassay technique (ELISA) adapted from the procedure described by Yolken and colleagues (10) was utilized. The commercially available kit termed Rotazyme was purchased from Abbott Laboratories, North Chicago, Illinois.

RESULTS

Comparison of Diarrhea to Virus Shedding

The relationship of rotavirus shedding to resolution of diarrhea in human infants is seen in Fig. 2. The mean duration of virus excretion in feces after onset of symptoms was approximately 11 days, with as little as 2 and as long as 30 days. A linear relationship between the resolution of diarrhea and cessation of viral shedding was observed. Generally, diarrhea stopped within 2 to 3 days of the end of viral shedding. Nearly identical data were obtained in mice (not shown). However, neither virus replication nor diarrhea exceeded 8 days after oral inoculation in the susceptible mice.

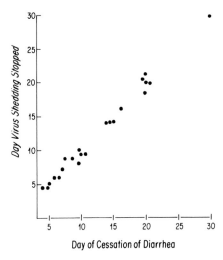

FIG. 2. Length of diarrhea compared with virus shedding. Each point represents one subject and depicts the day on which diarrhea resolved and the fecal sample was negative for rotavirus.

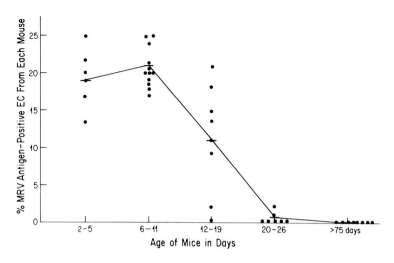

FIG. 3. Percent MRV-positive enterocytes isolated from the small intestine of infected and un-infected mice of varying ages.

Presence of MRV Antigen in Enterocytes 24 Hr After Oral Inoculation

The frequency of viral antigen positive cells appeared to be strictly age-dependent (Fig. 3). All of the mice aged 2 to 11 days, when inoculated, exhibited the presence of viral antigen in their enterocytes. The frequency of animals with virus-containing enterocytes was lower in those mice infected with virus at 12 to 29 days of age. No antigen positive cells were seen in mice infected after 26 days of age.

Enterocyte Binding of MRV

Susceptibility of enterocytes to MRV was measured by the ability to bind MRV-coated RBCs and produce rosettes. The distribution of enterocyte-binding to MRV-coated RBC, relative to the age of the mice at the time of collection of enterocytes, is presented in Fig. 4. The highest number of enterocytes with MRV-RBC rosettes was found in the suckling mice under 11 days of age. About 250 to 350 rosettes/2,000 enterocytes were observed in these animals. Subsequently, the number of such enterocytes declined with advancing age of the suckling mice and less than 75 to 100 virus-binding enterocytes were detected after 75 days of age. It is interesting to note that the temporal pattern of enterocyte-virus-binding *in vitro* was remarkably similar to the patterns of cytoplasmic viral antigen detected after *in vivo* infection of the intact animal. However, no antigen-positive enterocytes were observed in infected animals after 26 days of age, although small numbers of virus-binding enterocytes could

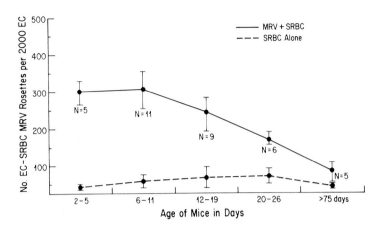

FIG. 4. Number of enterocyte-SRBC^{MRV} rosettes detected among enterocytes isolated from the small intestine of mice of varying age groups.

still be detected *in vitro* in this age group of animals, as well as in the older animals (after 75 days), as shown in Fig. 4.

COMMENTS

The association of rotavirus with the development of enteritis in human and other mammalian infants is well known. Our observations on the linear relationship between the shedding of virus and duration of the diarrhea suggest that the development of chronic diarrhea in some infants with rotavirus infection may be related to the continued viral replication. The alterations in cell-virus interaction in relationship to the severity of disease is also supported by changes in the development of virus-specific serum and secretory antibody response (7). Earlier studies from our laboratory have indicated that severe rotavirus infections with prolonged viral shedding is often associated with a reduced IgG rotavirus antibody response in the serum and an increased secretory IgA response in the feces (7).

In the present studies, an exquisite, age-related restriction of MRV-mouse enterocyte interaction was observed. This is evidenced by the presence of rotavirus antigen in only younger mice after induced infection in *in vivo* settings, and the binding of rotavirus to enterocytes of mice less than 75 days of age. These data suggest that the initial events in the attachment of rotavirus to the intestinal epithelium may be mediated by virus-specific receptors on villous enterocytes. It is possible that increased viral replication associated with disease may be related to the availability of much larger numbers of virus-specific receptors on the enterocytes in patients with severe disease than in patients with milder infections.

Based on the information presented in this report, it is not possible to determine the nature or mechanisms of induction of such receptors in the human intestine. However, several possible mechanisms may exist. The virus-binding receptors may represent sites similar to those previously identified of binding of immunoglobulin in the intestinal epithelium (5). It is also possible that environmental factors such as the host's hormonal milieu in infancy, prior bacterial or viral infection, etc. may regulate the induction and the magnitude of such binding sites.

In view of the fact that malnutrition greatly influences the mortality and morbidity of intense infections, it is tempting to postulate that the nutritional state of the host may play an important role in modulating the functional homeostasis and expression of virus-specific binding sites in the intestinal epithelium, and this determines the outcome of viral enteritis during malnutrition.

REFERENCES

1. Bishop, R. F., Davidson, G. P., Holmes, I. H., and Ruck, B. J. (1974): Detection of a new virus by electron microscopy of faecal extracts from children with acute gastroenteritis. *Lancet*, 1:149–151.
2. Davidson, G. P., Gall, D. G., Petric, M., Butler, D. G., and Hamilton, J. R. (1977): Human rotavirus enteritis induced in conventional piglets. *J. Clin. Invest.*, 60:1402–1407.
3. Kraft, L. M. (1957): Studies on the etiology and transmission of epidemic diarrhoea of infant mice. *J. Exp. Med.*, 101:743–755.
4. Mebus, C. A., Underdahl, N. R., Rhodes, M. B., and Twiehaus, M. J. (1969): Calf diarrhoea (scours): reproduced with a virus from a field outbreak. *University of Nebraska Agricultural Experiment Station Research Bulletin, No. 233.*
5. Nagura, H., Nakane, P. K., and Brown, W. R. (1978): Breast milk IgA binds to jejunal epithelium in suckling rats. *J. Immunol.*, 120:1333–1339.
6. Poston, R. N. (1974): A buffered chromium chloride method of attaching antigens to red cells: use in haemagglutination. *Immunol. Meth.*, 5:91–96.
7. Riepenhoff-Talty, M., Bogger-Goren, S., Li, P., Carmody, P., Barrett, H. J., and Ogra, P. L. (1981): Development of serum and intestinal antibody response to rotavirus after naturally acquired rotavirus infection in man. *J. Med. Virol.*, 8:215–222.
8. Weiser, M. M. (1973): Intestinal epithelial cell surface membrane glycoprotein synthesis. I. An indicator of cellular differentiation. *J. Biol. Chem.*, 248:2536–2541.
9. Woode, G. N., Bridger, J., Hall, G. A., Jones, J. M., and Jackson, G. (1976): The isolation of reovirus-like agents (rotavirus) from acute gastroenteritis of piglets. *J. Med. Microbiol.*, 9:203–209.
10. Yolken, R. H., Kim, H. W., Clem, T., Wyatt, R. G., Kalica, A. R., Chanock, R. M., and Kapikian, A. Z. (1977): Enzyme-linked immunosorbent assay (ELISA) for detection of human reovirus-like agent of infantile gastroenteritis. *Lancet*, 2:263–267.

Acute Diarrhea: Its Nutritional Consequences in Children, edited by J. A. Bellanti. Nestlé, Vevey/Raven Press, New York © 1983.

ETIOLOGIC AGENTS OF ACUTE DIARRHEA: VIRAL

Discussion

Dr. Kapikian: Recently, Dr. Masutto has been able to grow twenty out of twenty-four field isolates in cell cultures directly, and he has been able to show that these possibly fall into three sera types. This finding appears to show that there are perhaps a finite number of rotavirus sera types as in the rhinovirus field where there are over a hundred at present. Thus, the hopes of developing a vaccine are more plausible now because there are not literally hundreds of sera types.

The other approach that bears mentioning is one that is used by Dr. Greenberg in our laboratory. He took an uncultivable human rotavirus, co-infected cells with cultivable bovine virus, and by gene reassortment showed that he could get a cultivable strain. Also, at present, a third approach that has gained excitement in various circles around the world is the use of a heterotypic strain. For example, using the analogy of smallpox vaccination and taking an animal rotavirus, such as the bovine or the rhesus rotavirus that grows well in cell culture, and using this as a substitute in humans to see if this might be amenable to achieving protection. But, of course, those studies are still far off.

Concerning the presentation of Dr. Yolken, I was intrigued by the fact that 17% of the patients admitted to the hospital had adenovirus. This is quite different from other long-term studies that have been done, including those in Japan. I think it might be useful to put into perspective the respective roles of adenoviruses and rotaviruses. Rotaviruses, according to Dr. Yolken, were about 43%, which is what has been found in most studies around the world. But what is the reason for the high prevalence of adenoviruses in his studies?

Dr. Yolken: First, the population in our studies consisted of a large number of outpatients, which might be different from an inpatient population. Second, there is a very clear difference in the number of adenoviruses we have found over the last one or two years.

Dr. Kapikian: Dr. Brandt, you and your group have had a long and interesting association with adenoviruses. I wonder if you would care to comment or share any other additional information you might have.

Dr. Brandt: I might indicate we have some data and also, particularly last December, we saw somewhat of a change in the adenovirus. So possibly there may have been an unusual occurrence of adenovirus.

Dr. Kapikian: Type 38?

Dr. Brandt: They were viruses that could be visualized in the stool and probably at least four or five of those were adenoviruses. We studied 922 patients hospitalized for gastroenteritis and found that 36% of them had rotavirus, 5.1% had adenovirus, 2.3% had small, round particles in the general size of 27 nm. Altogether 43% of them had a virus that could be demonstrated by electron microscopy. We also had a group of control subjects who were hospitalized. Most had respiratory disease, and therefore from the standpoint of adenovirus we probably have a falsely high background. Of the hospitalized control group, 856 patients were studied; 2.1% had rotavirus, 2.08% adenovirus, 0.8% had 27 nm particles, and a total of 4.9% had a demonstrable virus. You will find that the overall totals do not precisely add up, and in these cases we are looking at dual infections. I might add that is something I think we should take a very hard look at. Over the years one-tenth of all the patients who had a rotavirus infection and were studied for a respiratory pathogen had, in fact, an isolable pathogen. I think a good deal of the diarrhea that has in the past been associated with influenza may, in fact, be a rotavirus and influenza infection occurring at the same time. In another study we looked at 299 outpatients with gastroenteritis; 20% had rotavirus, 3.7% adenovirus, 2.0% 27 nm particles, and 26.1% had a demonstrable virus by electron microscopy. In the 386 control subjects, 3.1% had rotavirus, 0.3% adenovirus, 0.5% 27 nm particles, and a total of 3.9% had a virus. I might add that we, too, have cultivated adenovirus. So far about 75% of our adenoviruses are enteric adenoviruses which respond to the enteroadenovirus antiserum. It is interesting to look at the enteric adenoviruses in relation to the patient's age. We studied 133 inpatients with gastroenteritis who were zero to 1 month of age; 1.5% were positive. Of 160 patients who were 2 to 3 months of age, 6.9% were adenovirus-positive. In the 4- to 5-month age group, 14 patients out of 104, i.e., 13.5%, were positive. In fact, that was the overall peak. In the 6- to 8-month age group, there were 5.2% positive; 9- to 12-month age group, 3.2%. There was a slight increase in the 13- to 18-month age group, 6.8%. Then in the 19- to 24-month group, 1.9% were positive. Equal to or greater than 25 months, 2.2% were positive for adenoviruses that could be visualized in the stool. So the adenoviruses had a tendency to peak earlier in life than the rotaviruses. Actually, they also peaked earlier in life than throat isolates. The peak for throat isolates in terms of percent of patients with an isolable adenovirus in this group was 6 to 8 months.

Dr. Bellanti: I think it is important to recall that adenoviruses have a propensity to the lymphoid tissue. Actually, this is where the viruses were originally isolated. The question also would arise as to whether these infections occurred in the presence of circulating antibodies. Did Dr. Brandt isolate adenovirus in the presence of serum antibody?

Dr. Brandt: We have not done a careful study of serum antibodies in most of these patients, so I cannot say. But looking at those who were 4 to 5 months of age, in a somewhat different way, I would suspect that we could demonstrate at least some form of adenovirus antibodies, but these would probably be antibodies from the mother.

Dr. Yolken: When we looked at our own data we had a very high rate of bacterial diarrhea in our urban populations. And we found a much higher rate of salmonella than was found in the initial hospital studies. Did you find any changes in the number of bacterial diarrhea in your population?

Dr. Brandt: There have been some changes with time. We have certainly seen instances of simultaneous viral and bacterial infection. We have also seen evidence of the simultaneous presence of rotavirus and adenovirus and rotavirus and 27 nm virus.

Acute Diarrhea: Its Nutritional Consequences in Children, edited by J. A. Bellanti.
Nestlé, Vevey/Raven Press, New York © 1983.

Etiologic Agents of Acute Diarrhea

Bacterial and Parasitic Agents of Acute Diarrhea

R. Bradley Sack

Division of Geographic Medicine, The Johns Hopkins University School of Medicine, Baltimore, Maryland 21224

The number of enteric bacteria recognized as causing acute diarrheal disease has increased rapidly during the past 10 years. Not only have new organisms been described, but new mechanisms of pathogenesis, including enterotoxin-mediated secretion, have been elucidated. Whereas previously very few (~20%) cases of acute diarrhea could be diagnosed etiologically, now that figure is closer to 80%, a large share being viral agents which have been discussed previously (33). It seems clear that new bacteriologic agents will also continue to be discovered in the years ahead, as research in this field continues. [Several studies of travelers have indicated that antibiotics can prevent diarrhea due to as yet unrecognized agents (31,32).] Also, it seems clear that the present methodology for making bacterial diagnoses will be simplified in the years to come, so that most laboratories will eventually have these capabilities. At present, the "80% success rate" in diagnosis applies only to those laboratories with the most advanced technology.

The present chapter is not meant to be exhaustive. A number of reviews recently have been published which deal with this subject in greater detail (7,9,11,30). Rather, this chapter will attempt to summarize our present state of knowledge, and will indicate where it is particularly sparse.

ORGANISMS CAUSING ACUTE DIARRHEA

The bacterial and parasitic pathogens to be discussed appear in Table 1. The organisms have been listed according to their primary pathogenetic mechanism: invasion or enterotoxin production. As will be noted, there is a column indicating that some mechanisms are as yet unknown; some of these may include intense mucosal colonization which has not yet been fully characterized.

Only two protozoa are included in Table 1; these are by far the most common. However, it is known that some parasites cause diarrhea in immuno-compromised hosts primarily (such as *Strongyloides stercoralis*) or only when

TABLE 1. *Recognized bacterial and parasitic causes of acute diarrheal disease*

Enterotoxigenic	Invasive	Unknown mechanisms
Vibrio cholerae 01	Shigella	Vibrio parahemolyticus
Vibrio cholerae NON 01 (NAGS)	Salmonella	Aeromonas hydrophila
Escherichia coli	Escherichia coli	Giardia lamblia
Clostridium perfringens	Staphylococcus aureus	
Bacillus cereus	Yersinia enterocolitica	
Staphylococcus aureus	Campylobacter jejuni	
Clostridium difficile	Entamoeba histolytica	

large worm loads are present (such as *Strongyloides, Trichuris trichiura*) and others much less common (such as *Balantidium coli*).

LABORATORY DIAGNOSIS

The diagnosis is primarily one of identifying the bacteria or parasite in the acute stool specimen. Although retrospective serologic diagnosis is possible with some of the agents, this is only of epidemiologic usefulness, since the illness will have resolved by the time this diagnosis is made.

Gross Examination

Gross examination of the stool can sometimes be of use in categorizing the etiologic agent. The presence of obvious blood and/or purulence suggests that an invasive organism is involved. On the other hand, a watery appearance with only small amounts of fecal material suggests that an enterotoxigenic organism is involved. In the majority of cases, however, the stool characteristics alone will not be diagnostic.

Direct Microscopic Examination

Direct microscopic examination can also be helpful to differentiate invasive from enterotoxigenic type illness, and, of course, for the recognition of protozoa and larger parasites. The presence of large numbers of pus cells (as seen by methylene blue stain) suggests an invasive etiology; the absence of large numbers of pus cells does not rule this out, however. In noninvasive disease, few or no pus cells are seen. An ordinary gram stain of stool is of limited usefulness, and is not recommended as a routine diagnostic procedure. A dark field examination of stool may be useful in recognizing the characteristic darting motility of the vibrios (2) (which can be immobilized by specific antisera), or the characteristic appearance of *Campylobacter* (24). Fluorescence antibody microscopy can be useful in some circumstances (*V. cholerae*, certain serotypes of *Escherichia coli*) but this procedure has never been widely adapted, probably due to its relative insensitivity, and because of the large numbers of serotypes of enteric pathogens being searched for.

Cultural Diagnosis

Cultural diagnosis is the most widely used method for recognition of bacterial pathogens. Usual enteric media can be used for isolation of *Shigella*, *Salmonella*, *Yersinia*, and *Aeromonas*. On the other hand, highly selective media have been devised for some organisms [such as thiosulfate citrate bile salts (TCBS) media for *V. cholerae* and *V. parahemolyticus* and Campy agar or its equivalent for *Campylobacter*, which is incubated at 42°C]. A recent review should be consulted for details of these examinations (33).

In some diarrheas of bacterial origin, such as "food poisoning" due to *Bacillus cereus*, *Staphylococcus aureus*, or *Clostridium perfringens*, the organisms cannot be cultured readily from the stool; rather, culture of the food is the important diagnostic maneuver.

In the case of *E. coli* diagnosis, one cannot differentiate a colony of normal *E. coli* from one that is diarrheagenic. Therefore, one has to test for the production of enterotoxins by these strains, or identify them serotypically (as will be discussed later) in order to establish them as etiologically related to the diarrhea.

Other Diagnostic Methods

Other diagnostic methods include recognition of toxins in the stools, such as in *Clostridium difficile*- or *E. coli*-mediated disease (8,19), or recognition of specific DNA sequences by probe techniques, as in the case of *V. cholerae*- and *E. coli*-mediated disease (20). These newer techniques, though limited to research laboratories at present, may eventually be simplified to the point of widespread application.

PATHOGENESIS AND PATHOPHYSIOLOGY

By far the best understood mechanism of pathogenesis is that which involves the hosts' response to enterotoxin production by bacteria growing in the small bowel (29). Less well understood is the mechanism of invasion by virulent organisms growing in the distal bowel.

Secretory Diarrheas

Those diarrheal illnesses mediated through the production of enterotoxins are termed secretory diarrheas. In this type of illness, the organisms are ingested by mouth (usually fairly large numbers are necessary, 10^{5-10} organisms) and must pass through the acid environment of the stomach into the normally almost sterile small bowel, where they attach to the mucosa by means of lectins or fimbria (CFA I and II in human *E. coli*). There they grow to large concentrations (10^{6-8} organisms/g tissue), and produce enterotoxins which attach to specific binding sites on the epithelial cells. The mechanism of attachment and biochemical events best studied are those related to *V. cholerae* enterotoxin. It is known that GM_1, ganglioside present in the epithelial cell membrane, is a receptor for the binding B subunit of the *V. cholerae* enterotoxin molecule. The B subunit, having attached to this receptor, remains in/on the membrane, while the active A subunit is transported into the cell where it brings about the activation of adenylate cyclase leading to an increase in cyclic adenosine monophosphate (cyclic AMP). This further leads to active chloride hypersecretion by the cell, and to a lesser extent, inhibition of sodium absorption by the cell. These biochemical effects result in the outpouring of large amounts of electrolyte-rich fluid into the small bowel, which overcomes the capacity of the rest of the distal bowel to absorb it, thus leading to watery diarrhea (10,14).

The heat-labile enterotoxin of *E. coli* is very closely related biochemically and antigenically to that of *V. cholerae*, and appears to act on the cell almost identically. The heat-stable enterotoxin, on the other hand, is a quite different molecule, nonantigenic and much smaller in size, and does not activate adenylate cyclase, but rather guanylate cyclase with resultant increases in cyclic guanosine monophosphate (cyclic GMP). *Yersinia enterocolitica*, only when grown at low temperature, produces a heat-stable enterotoxin similar, if not identical, to that of *E. coli* (22), but there is no suggestion that the enterotoxin is involved in disease. Similarly, strains of *Salmonella* produce a *V. cholerae*-like enterotoxin (25), whose role in the pathogenesis of diarrhea is still not fully understood. *Shigella* organisms also produce a cytotoxic enterotoxin which has been well characterized and is thought to mediate some features of the invasive-type illness, although this, too, is not well understood (23). Other organisms that produce enterotoxins are listed in Table 1. The best understood of these are those produced by *C. difficile*, the primary etiologic agent of antibiotic-related pseudomembranous enterocolitis. These enterotoxins are causally related to the diarrheal disease induced by the large numbers of organisms growing in the large intestine (1).

The genetic material which codes for the production of enterotoxin may be located in plasmids (as in the case of *E. coli*) or in the chromosome (as in *V. cholerae*). Having the enterotoxin-mediating genes in transferable elements is undoubtedly of importance (as yet not fully worked out) in the transmission of the organism and the related diseases.

Invasive Diarrheas

Much less is understood of the mechanism whereby invasive diarrheas are caused. The responsible organisms, also ingested by mouth (usually lower inocula are required), must escape the acid environment of the stomach, traverse most of the small bowel before they colonize the terminal ileum or large bowel, and invade the mucosa there. What allows the organisms to enter the mucosal cells is not known. In some organisms, such as *Yersinia*, the presence of plasmids has been associated with this invasive ability, although exactly what enzymes or related substances are involved is not clear (36).

Once invasion occurs, an intense inflammatory reaction takes place in the host, resulting in the outpouring of pus cells, and sometimes blood, in the diarrheal stool. The organisms may occasionally invade the blood stream and cause bacteremia in the host which adds to the toxic, clinical picture of the disease.

In both secretory and invasive diarrheas, the disease is self-limiting, probably because of the immune mechanisms of the host. This usually occurs in 1 to 7 days, probably reflecting the prior immunologic experience of the host. It is known that antibody-producing plasma cells in the lamina propria produce specific IgA secretory antibody which can be measured in the lumen. The appearance of these specific cells in the gut is an immunologic marker of the protection of the host against a particular organism/antigen (27).

The pathogenetic mechanisms involved in protozoal-mediated diarrheas are even less well understood. Certain virulent *Entamoeba histolytica* strains have been found to have a specific isoenzyme pattern that may distinguish them from nonpathogenic strains. Also some strains have been shown to produce "enterotoxins" that could be involved in the disease process (18).

EPIDEMIOLOGY

All of the bacterial and parasitic causes of acute diarrhea are spread by the fecal-oral route, usually through contaminated food or water. Where this transmission occurs with high frequency, the incidence of these diseases is high (35). In all geographic areas, however, acute diarrheal diseases are overwhelmingly a disease of young children, primarily between the ages of 6 months to 2 years. Following repeated episodes of diarrhea and/or infection, children become immune to most of the prevalent pathogens, and the disease rate drops precipitously. If into this environment, however, come immunologically-naive adults, such as travelers from the developed world, acute diarrhea occurs with a very high attack rate, and the organisms responsible are the same as those which cause disease in the small children (31,32). Adult travelers also have a markedly decreased attack rate if they remain in the area for prolonged periods of time.

In only a few areas have extensive etiologically-related epidemiologic studies been done. In these studies (3), enterotoxigenic *E. coli* are found to be the most frequent pathogens in the very young, although they usually cause relatively mild disease. Rotavirus, by way of contrast, more often causes severe disease, but is less frequent. This observation probably relates to the multiple virulence antigens found in enterotoxigenic *E. coli*, a noninvasive organism, and the few serotypes of rotavirus which is, by definition, an invasive pathogen.

Relatively less is known of the other bacterial pathogens. Some, such as *Yersinia* and *Campylobacter*, are known to be frequent in certain animal species, and animal-to-human transmission is undoubtedly important. Some organisms, like vibrios, are related to marine environment and are transmitted to man through ingestion of shellfish.

SPECIFIC ORGANISMS

Some additional, particularly applicable information will be added about specific bacteria.

V. cholerae

V. cholerae is the only one of the bacterial agents that has been responsible for true pandemic disease. (We are currently in the seventh pandemic.) Although thought initially to be entirely a human organism, there is now evidence that shellfish or marine environments alone may be reservoirs for this organism (4). This has been particularly noted since the recent cholera outbreaks in the United States and Australia.

The enterotoxin produced by *V. cholerae* has been the most widely studied of all the enterotoxins, and remains the prototype.

E. coli

E. coli have been found to produce diarrheal disease by at least one additional mechanism in animals, that of heavy colonization of the mucosa, without specific enterotoxin production or invasion (6). The most common diarrhea-related strains are enterotoxigenic, and they occur primarily in the developing world where sanitation is poor. Invasive *E. coli* occur much less commonly; they produce an illness indistinguishable from shigellosis. Such organisms share antigens with *Shigella* and may be confused with them on primary isolation.

Enteropathogenic *E. coli* are specific serotypes of *E. coli* (such as serogroups 0111, 055) which are known to cause outbreaks of diarrhea, primarily in newborns. Although they do not produce the enterotoxins that enterotoxigenic *E. coli* produce, they seem to produce other enterotoxins which have not yet been well characterized (17). Whether all serotypes of *E. coli* called "enteropathogenic" are indeed that, particularly when isolated from sporadic cases of diarrhea, is under much doubt, at present.

In the case of an outbreak of diarrhea thought to be due to *E. coli*, both serotype and enterotoxin production should be characterized to define an etiologic role.

Campylobacter jejuni

Campylobacter jejuni is an organism that is assuming increasing importance in our understanding of the bacterial diarrheas, particularly as selective media and growth conditions are now available for routine laboratory studies. *Campylobacter* probably accounts for 2 to 8% of acute diarrheal episodes, similar in frequency to that of *Salmonella* and *Shigella*. This organism has been isolated from young dogs and other animals, and these may be a reservoir of infection. In some parts of the world, high carrier rates (35%) are found in children, and it is difficult to associate the organism with a particular disease episode (5).

The disease syndrome is not usually specific, but may include bloody diarrhea as a prominent feature. Although some antibiotics show *in vivo* effectiveness, there is still no demonstrated, clear, clinical effect of antibiotics on the course of this disease.

Yersinia enterocolitica

Yersinia enterocolitica is also animal-related, and several outbreaks have been traced to contaminated milk. They are easily isolated from diarrheal stools, and cold enrichment is not necessary to diagnose clinical cases. Only a few serotypes are thought to be pathogenic; others are frequently isolated from the environment (34). These organisms seem to be rarely isolated from sporadic cases of diarrhea, and are more apt to be recognized as outbreak-related.

Aeromonas hydrophila and *Plesiomonas shigelloides*

Both *Aeromonas hydrophila* and *Plesiomonas shigelloides* are recently reported agents that may be important in the causation of diarrhea. Both produce enterotoxins, as yet not well characterized. It is not known how important these organisms are in the full spectrum of pathogens.

C. difficile

C. difficile is the causative agent of antibiotic-related pseudomembranous enterocolitis and is best recognized by the presence of the cytoxin(s) it produces in stool samples. Although the disease occasionally occurs unrelated to antibiotic administration, it has not been found important in the usual acute diarrhea syndromes (*unpublished data*).

V. parahemolyticus

Disease caused by *V. parahemolyticus* is primarily related to ingestion of raw seafood. The mechanism whereby this organism causes diarrhea is not well understood, though in some circumstances it produces both an invasive or a secretory type illness. It is a common marine organism, which grows to large concentrations during the warm weather.

V. cholerae non-01

V. cholerae non-01, the so-called nonagglutinating vibrios or NAGs, are associated with both sporadic cases and outbreaks of diarrheal illness. Some strains produce an enterotoxin indistinguishable from that of *V. cholerae* 01 (37); the mechanism by which the remaining organisms produce illness is not known.

Shigella

The *Shigella* organisms are noted for the low inoculum required to cause illness, often as few as 10 to 100 organisms. Although primarily invasive, they produce an enterotoxin which has now been purified and characterized, and which may be important in initiating the disease process. The illness produced by these organisms may involve considerable protein loss in the stool, and thus may be of particular importance in poorly nourished children.

Although easily recognizable when growing on enteric media, the organisms are often difficult to culture from stool, even from known cases.

Salmonella

Nontyphoidal salmonellae are of greater importance as diarrhea-causing agents in the developed world than in the developing world. This seems to be related to food-processing techniques that assist in their dissemination. Although there are large numbers of serotypes, only a few are responsible for most diarrheal disease in any specific area. Antibiotics have not been shown to be of value in treating diarrheal illness due to these organisms, and they may prolong the carrier state (21). For this reason, they should only be used when systemic disease is suspected or confirmed.

Clostridium perfringens

Enterotoxin-producing strains are responsible for large numbers of food-related diarrheal episodes. The enterotoxin is released during sporulation of the organisms following ingestion. The disease is usually mild; diagnosis can be made only from examination of the food ingested, or in retrospective serologic diagnosis, based on antitoxins in serum.

Certain strains of the organism are also responsible for pigbel in the New Guinea highlands, in which the organisms invade and proliferate in the small bowel. This is postulated to be due to a decrease in small intestinal proteases brought about by a diet low in protein and rich in sweet potato, which contains trypsin inhibitors; this situation then allows the beta toxin of *C. perfringens* type C to initiate the disease (16). The disease can be prevented by immunization with the specific toxoid of the organism (15).

Staphylococcus aureus

Staphylococcal "food poisoning," one of the earliest recognized enterotoxigenic diseases, results from the ingestion of preformed enterotoxin in food.

This enterotoxin has primarily a central nervous system effect and is quite different from the other enterotoxins discussed.

Invasive staphylococci have been incriminated in antibiotic-related pseudomembranous enterocolitis, but seem to be of much less importance than *C. difficile.*

Bacillus cereus

B. cereus is also a cause of food poisoning; two clinical syndromes (predominantly vomiting or diarrhea) develop depending on the type of enterotoxin produced, and whether the enterotoxin is present in the ingested food. Diagnosis can usually be made only in outbreaks, and only by examining the suspect foods.

Giardia lamblia

Giardia lamblia seems to produce acute diarrheal disease in nonimmune individuals, whereas asymptomatic carriage of the organism is much more common. The gelatin capsule string test has made the sampling of duodenal contents relatively easy, thus improving diagnostic capabilities.

Other Organisms

Reports of other bacteria being related to acute diarrhea have been made, but a causal relationship is yet to be established. These organisms include *Pseudomonas, Klebsiella, Proteus, Enterobacter*; some of these have also been shown to produce enterotoxins (12,13).

THERAPY OF ACUTE DIARRHEAL DISEASES

There are three main aspects of therapy of all the described diseases: (a) replacement of fluid and electrolytes lost in the stool, (b) maintenance of nutrition by early feeding, and (c) use of appropriate antibiotics when indicated.

The most important aspect of therapy is to replace diarrheal losses so that the normal physiology of the body can be maintained. When the losses are severe, the replacement must be made by the intravenous route, at least initially. Several solutions can be used; one satisfactory solution is Ringer's lactate. If the losses are moderate or mild, or following the initial intravenous replacement of losses in severe dehydration, the replacement can be given orally in nearly all cases. This is true regardless of the etiology of the diarrhea (viral or bacterial) and regardless of the age of the patient. A universal diarrheal replacement solution has been developed by the World Health Organization (WHO) which has proved satisfactory in both the developing world and in developed countries. This is based on the observation that active glucose absorption in the small bowel, which is largely intact in acute diarrheal diseases, will facilitate sodium absorption, on roughly a 1:1 basis (1 mmol glucose will facilitate the absorption of 1 mmol sodium). The composition is given in Table 2. The only limitations to the use of the solution are (a) a high stool rate (>10 ml/kg/hr) as may be seen occasionally in cholera, (b) intractable vomiting, seen in <1% of children, although most children have some vomiting as part of their illness, and (c) occasional glucose intolerance, also seen in <1% of children; if glucose is not absorbed, sodium will also not be absorbed (26,28). This therapy has been successfully employed in hospitals, clinics, and homes, and forms the backbone of the WHO global diarrhea control program.

The second important aspect of therapy is to provide food supplements to the child as soon as possible, to avoid the adverse nutritional consequences of the disease. Food can be given as early as 8 hr after the beginning of therapy. Breast-feeding should be maintained, with only a few hours' interruption during the early phases of therapy.

Antibiotics are useful only in a few of the diarrheal illnesses due to bacteria (see Table 3). From a clinical standpoint, antibiotics are used only (a) if there is a strong clinical suspicion of cholera in a cholera endemic area, or (b) if the clinical picture suggests invasive disease, such as shigellosis, (c) if the child is clinically toxic and systemic salmonellosis is suspected, or (d) if pseudomembranous enterocolitis is diagnosed clinically. In the vast majority of cases, then, no antibiotics are indicated (7).

Specific therapy is available for diarrhea due to giardiasis and amebiasis, and will lead to clinical improvement and shortening of the disease. It should be noted that particularly with *Giardia*, infection may recur, and not necessarily be associated with clinical illness.

PREVENTION

Preventing diarrheal illness depends on interrupting transmission by environmental means, or protecting the host by immunologic mechanisms. The

TABLE 2. *Composition of oral glucose-electrolyte solution used for therapy of acute diarrheal diseases[a]*

	mmol/liter
Sodium	90
Potassium	20
Chloride	80
Bicarbonate	30
Glucose	111

[a] One liter contains sodium chloride, 3.5 g; sodium bicarbonate, 2.5 g; potassium chloride, 1.5 g; glucose, 20.0 g, or sucrose, 40.0 g.

TABLE 3. *Antimicrobial agents in acute diarrheal disease*

Therapeutics	Drugs
Established therapeutic value	Drugs of choice
Cholera	Tetracycline, furazolidone
Shigellosis	Ampicillin, trimethoprim-sulfamethoxazole
	(others, depending on sensitivity testing)
Antibiotic-related pseudomembranous	
enterocolitis	Vancomycin
Amebiasis	Metranidazole
Giardiasis	Quinacrine hydrochloride
Uncertain therapeutic value	Drugs of possible value
Enterotoxigenic *Escherchia coli*	Tetracycline
Campylobacter jejuni	Erythromycin, tetracycline
Yersinia enterocolitica	Tetracycline, trimethoprim-sulfamethoxazole
No therapeutic value	
Nontyphoid salmonellosis	
Uncomplicated viral diarrheas	
Prophylactic value	Drugs of choice
Travellers' diarrhea (enterotoxigenic	Doxycycline, trimethoprim-sulfamethoxazole,
E. coli)	tetracycline
Cholera, short term, close contacts	

former is by far the most effective, but is beyond the immediate means of most of the developing world. Immunologic control is therefore an important research area at the present time. Live attenuated *V. cholerae* and enterotoxic *E. coli* vaccines are being developed in the laboratory and may prove useful in the field. Both are based on the concept that stimulation of the local immune response of the gut should afford the maximal protection against subsequent diarrheal illness.

FUTURE WORK

The most pressing problem is to find ways to make effective therapy available to all persons with acute diarrhea, on a world-wide basis. WHO and other national and international agencies are using oral therapy to accomplish this and it should result in a marked decrease in diarrhea-related mortality. Work is also going on to define pharmacologic agents that might stop the diarrhea, thus markedly shortening the disease and making therapy even easier to administer. New bacterial agents have yet to be recognized, and the pathogenetic mechanisms of many of the known organisms have not yet been worked out. Studies of how to optimally immunize the gastrointestinal tract with the most appropriate antigens may lead to a decrease in diarrhea attack-rates and morbidity. Epidemiology studies are being done to define populations whose diarrheagenic agents are defined, so that appropriate field trials of vaccine may be done. Finally, methods of interrupting transmission of pathogens are being studied, even before the final solution of good water, sewerage, and education can be widely implemented.

REFERENCES

1. Bartlett, J. G. (1979): Antibiotic-associated pseudomembranous colitis. *Rev. Infect. Dis.*, 1:530.
2. Benenson, A. S., Islam, M. R., Greenough III, W. B. (1964): Rapid identification of *Vibrio cholerae* by darkfield microscopy. *Bull. WHO*, 30:827–831.
3. Black, R. E., Merson, M. H., Rahman, A. S. M. M., Yunus, M., Alim, A. R. M. A., Huq, I., Yolken, R. H., and Curlin, G. T. (1980): A two-year study of bacterial, viral, and parasitic agents associated with diarrhea in rural Bangladesh. *J. Infect. Dis.*, 142:660–664.
4. Blake, P. A., Allegra, D. T., Snyder, J. D., Barrett, T. J., McFarland, L., Caraway, C. T., Feeley, J. C., Craig, J. P., Lee, J. V., Puhr, N. D., Feldman, R. A. (1980): Cholera—a possible focus in the United States. *N. Engl. J. Med.*, 302:305–309.
5. Blaser, M. J., and Reller, L. B. (1981): Campylobacter enteritis. *N. Engl. J. Med.*, 305:1444–1451.
6. Cantey, J. R., and Blake, R. K. (1977): Diarrhea due to *Escherichia coli* in the rabbit: a novel mechanism. *J. Infect. Dis.*, 135:454–462.
7. Carpenter, C. C. J., and Sack, R. B. (1981): Infectious diarrheal syndromes. *In: Harrison's Principles of Internal Medicine*, 9th ed., pp. 209–229. McGraw-Hill, New York.
8. Chang, T-W., Lauermann, M., and Bartlett, J. G. (1979): Cytotoxicity assay in antibiotic-associated colitis. *J. Infect. Dis.*, 140:765–770.
9. Holme, T., Holmgren, J., Merson, M. H., and Mollby, R. (editors) (1981): Acute enteric infections in children. New prospects for treatment and prevention. *Proceedings of the 3rd Nobel Conference, Stockholm*. Elsevier/North-Holland, Amsterdam.
10. Holmgren, J. (1981): Actions of cholera toxin and the prevention and treatment of cholera. *Nature*, 292:413–417.
11. Keusch, G. T. (1979): Shigella infections. *Clin. Gastroenterol.*, 8:645.
12. Klipstein, F. A., Engert, R. F., and Short, H. B. (1977): Relative enterotoxigenicity of coliform bacteria. *J. Infect. Dis.*, 136:205–215.
13. Kubota, Y., and Liu, P. V. (1971): An enterotoxin of *Pseudomonas aeruginosa. J. Infect. Dis.*, 123:97–98.
14. Lai, C-Y. (1980): The chemistry and biology of cholera toxin. *Crit. Rev. Biochem.*, 9:171–206.
15. Lawrence, G., Shann, F., Freestone, D. S., and Walker, P. D. (1979): Prevention of necrotising enteritis in Papua New Guinea by active immunisation. *Lancet*, i:266–267.
16. Lawrence, G., and Walker, P. D. (1976): Pathogenesis of enteritis necroticans in Papua New Guinea. *Lancet*, i:125–126.
17. Levine, M. M., Nalin, D. R., Hornick, R. B., Bergquist, E. J., Waterman, D. H., Young, E. R., and Sotman, S. (1978): *Escherichia coli* strains that cause diarrhea but do not produce heat-labile or heat-stable enterotoxins and are noninvasive. *Lancet*, i:1119–1122.
18. Lushbaugh, W. B., Kairalla, A. B., Cantey, J. R., Hofbauer, A. F., and Pittman, F. E. (1979): Isolation of a cytotoxin-enterotoxin from *Entamoeba histolytica. J. Infect. Dis.*, 139:9–17.
19. Merson, M. H., Yolken, R. H., Sack, R. B., Froehlich, J. L., Greenberg, H. B., Huq, I., and Black, R. W. (1980): Detection of *Escherichia coli* enterotoxins in stools. *Infect. Immun.*, 29:108–113.
20. Moseley, S. L., Huq, I., Alim, A. R. M. A., So, M., Samadpour-Motalebi, M., and Falkow, S. (1980): Detection of enterotoxigenic *Escherichia coli* by DNA colony hybridization. *J. Infect. Dis.*, 142:892–898.
21. Nelson, J. D., Kusmiesz, H., Jackson, L. H., and Woodman, E. (1980): Treatment of *Salmonella* gastroenteritis with ampicillin, amoxicillin, or placebo. *Pediatrics*, 65:1125–1130.
22. Okamoto, K., Inque, T., Ichikawa, H., Kawamoto, Y., and Myama, A. (1981): Partial purification and characterization of heat-stable enterotoxin produced by *Yersinia enterocolitica. Infect. Immun.*, 31:554–559.
23. Olsnes, S., and Eiklid, K. (1980): Isolation and characterization of *Shigella shigae* cytotoxin. *J. Biol. Chem.*, 255:284–289.
24. Paisley, J. W., Mirrett, S., Lauer, B. A., Roe, M., and Reller, L. B. (1982): Darkfield microscopy of human feces for presumptive diagnosis of *Campylobacter-fetus* subsp. *jejuni* enteritis. *J. Clin. Microbiol.*, 15:61–63.
25. Peterson, J. W. (1980): Salmonella toxin. *Pharmacol. Ther.*, 11:719–724.
26. Pierce, N. F., and Hirschhorn, N. (1977): Oral fluid—a simple weapon against dehydration in diarrhea: how it works and how to use it. *WHO Chronicle*, 31(3):87–93.

27. Pierce, N. F., and Sack, R. B. (1977): Immune response of the intestinal mucosa to cholera toxoid. *J. Infect. Dis.*, 136:S113–S117.
28. Population Reports (1980): Oral rehydration therapy (ORT) for childhood diarrhea. *Population Information Program, The Johns Hopkins University*, Series L, No. 2.
29. Robins-Browne, R. M. (1980): Enterotoxins and disease. *S. Afr. J. Sci.*, 76:352–359.
30. Sack, R. B. (1980): Enterotoxigenic *Escherichia coli* identification and characterization. *J. Infect. Dis.*, 142:279–286.
31. Sack, R. B., Froehlich, J. L., Zulich, A. W., Sidi Hidi, D., Kapikian, A. Z., Orskov, F., Orskov, I., and Greenberg, H. B. (1979): Prophylactic doxycycline for travelers' diarrhea: results of a prospective double-blind study of Peace Corps Volunteers in Morocco. *Gastroenterology*, 76:1368–1373.
32. Sack, R. B., Santosham, M., Froehlich, J. L., Medina, C., Orskov, F., and Orskov, I. (1982): Daily doxycycline prevents travelers' diarrhea in Honduras, an area where resistance to doxycycline is common among enterotoxigenic *Escherichia coli. J. Infect. Dis. (submitted).*
33. Sack, R. B. (1981): Diagnosis of enterotoxigenic *Escherichia coli* infections. In: *Acute Enteric Infections in Children. New Prospects for Treatment and Prevention*, edited by T. Holme, J. Holmgren, M. H. Merson, and R. Molby. Elsevier/North-Holland Biomedical Press, Amsterdam.
34. Schielmann, D. A., and Devenish, J. A. (1982): Relationship of HeLa cell infectivity to biochemical, serological, and virulence characteristics of *Yersinia enterocolitica. Infect. Immun.*, 35:497–506.
35. Woodward, W. E., Hirschhorn, N., Sack, R. B., Cash, R. A., Brownlee, I., Chickadonz, G. H., Evans, L. K., Shepard, R. H., and Woodward, R. C. (1974): Acute diarrhea on an Apache Indian reservation. *Am. J. Epidemiol.*, 99:281–290.
36. Zink, D. L., Feeley, J. C., Wells, J. G., Vanderzant, G., Vickery, J. C., Roof, W. D., and O'Donovan, G. A. (1980): Plasmid-mediated tissue invasiveness in *Yersinia enterocolitica. Nature (Lond.)*, 283:224–226.
37. Zinnaka, Y., and Carpenter, Jr., C. C. J. (1972): An enterotoxin produced by noncholera vibrios. *Johns Hopkins Med. J.*, 131:403–411.

Acute Diarrhea: Its Nutritional Consequences in Children, edited by J. A. Bellanti.
Nestlé, Vevey/Raven Press, New York © 1983.

Etiologic Agents of Acute Diarrhea: Bacterial and Parasitic

Comments

Guillermo Ruiz-Palacios

Infectious Diseases Department, National Institute of Nutrition, Tlalpan, Mexico 22, D.F., Mexico

Dr. Sack has masterly summarized the present state of knowledge on the etiology of acute diarrhea, making it possible to concentrate on some aspects that I consider relevant.

ETIOLOGIC AGENTS IN DIFFERENT POPULATIONS

The frequency of agents causing acute diarrhea will differ depending on the type of population studied, and one should ask, where am I? and what age am I studying? Table 1 compiles recent information on etiologic agents associated with diarrheal illnesses in the community from developing and developed countries in children under 2 years of age (2,3,10). Here we can see the striking similarity of the frequency of etiologic agents when populations are compared on the basis of the quality of sanitation, rather than geographic location.

Enterotoxigenic *E. coli* (ETEC), rotavirus (RV) and *Campylobacter* (CFJ) represent more than half of all the causes of diarrhea in developing countries. Therefore, any attempt at prevention of acute diarrhea in the community, such as the development of vaccines or interruption of transmission cycles, should be oriented mainly against these three organisms. This is not true for developed countries, where RV, *Shigella*, and *Salmonella* are the predominant agents.

In contrast to what happens in the community, 30 to 50% of the children with diarrhea admitted to a hospital, regardless of the country, are infected with RV (6,9).

ADHERENCE FACTORS

The colonization is the first event in the pathogenesis of bacteria whose door of entry is the mucosa, as in ETEC and *Vibrio cholerae*. It is generally, but not always, mediated by pili, and in the same way can be detected by the property to agglutinate erythrocytes of different animal species in presence of

TABLE 1. *Etiologic agents of acute diarrhea in children in the community in developing and developed countries*[a]

	Developing			Developed	
	Bangladesh[b]	Brazil[c]	Mexico[d]	Canada[e]	USA[f]
Enterotoxigenic *Escherichia coli*	20	22	21	1	4
Rotavirus	11	19	18	11	10
Campylobacter	NI	11	15	NI	NI
Shigella	15	8	5	11	25
Salmonella	NS	—	1	1.4	2
Giardia	NS	6.7	2	NI	4
Yersinia	NS	—	2	NI	NI
Entamoeba histolytica	NS	2	2	NI	—
Aeromonas	NS	1	1	NI	NI
Plesiomonas	NS	—	1	NI	NI

NI = not investigated; NS = not specified.
[a] Children under 2 years of age.
[b] From ref. 2.
[c] From ref. 13.
[d] From ref. 11.
[e] From ref. 5.
[f] From ref. 10.

mannose. When CFA/I and II were identified, it was thought that these were the only, or more important, antigens associated with adhesion of ETEC. But things have proven to be more complex. Epidemiologic studies looking for these adherence traits, summarized in Table 2, have shown that:

1. In approximately half of the enterotoxigenic strains it has not been possible to demonstrate adherence factors.
2. CFA/I and II are not the only colonization factors.
3. Even though the erythrocyte agglutination is a good test for screening, there are enterotoxigenic strains that do not produce any type of hemagglutination, but possess fimbria and adhere, as proven in the baby rabbit model (15).
4. There are some enteropathogenic strains which do not produce enterotoxins and do not possess pili, but heavily colonize the intestine inducing diarrhea (3,14).

TABLE 2. *Frequency of adherence factors in ETEC strains*

Reference	No. strains	CFA/I	CFA/II	Others	No adherence
Cravioto (4)	187	17	25	—	—
Bergman (1)	40	20	2.5	17.5	60
Ruiz-Palacios[d]	17[a]	12	35	17	35
Ruiz-Palacios[d]	19[b]	15	5	37[c]	44

[a] Adult travelers.
[b] Children.
[c] Twenty-six percent belong to CFA/V.
[d] Unpublished data.

Thus, what looked like a rather simple approach to vaccination against ETEC with the pili requires further work on characterization of new pili and better knowledge of the prevalence of these antigens in different geographic areas. But since these antigens are plasmid-regulated, the task can become even more difficult to achieve if strains show periodic shifts.

CAMPYLOBACTER

There is no doubt that CFJ is an important cause of diarrhea throughout the world, but there are several questions yet to be answered. Does the isolation of CFJ necessarily implicate it as the causal agent? Does CFJ possess, as *E. coli* does, virulence factors such as the ability to invade or the ability to produce enterotoxins?

We have shown in experimental models that CFJ is, indeed, an invasive organism (12). But when we tried different strains isolated from patients with diarrhea, not all of them induced the disease in chicken. Clinically, it has been observed that only 20% of the cases of CFJ diarrhea are associated with fecal leukocytes, and the clinical picture resembles that of a secretory diarrhea thus suggesting that CFJ can produce toxins.

We have very recently demonstrated in 30% of the strains the presence of two types of enterotoxins (11). Their production is induced only by the addition of serine to the media at a concentration of 0.25% as in the case of *V. cholerae* and *V. parahaemolyticus* (7,8). Some strains on VERO (African green monkey kidney cells) and CHO (Chinese hamster ovary cells) have a cytolytic effect, and others a cytopathic effect (elongation), similar to the one described for cholera toxin and heat-stable toxin of ETEC. There are strains that show both effects. Most of these strains also induce fluid secretion in the rat ileal loop but not in rabbit.

REFERENCES

1. Bergman, M. J., Updike, W. S., Wood, S. J. et al. (1981): Attachment factors among enterotoxigenic *Escherichia coli* from patients with acute diarrhea from diverse geographic areas. *Infect. Immun.*, 32:881–888.
2. Black, R. E., Merson, M. H., Huq, I., Alim, A. R., and Yunus, M. D. (1981): Incidence and severity of rotavirus and *Escherichia coli* diarrhea in rural Bangladesh. Implication for vaccine development. *Lancet*, 1:141–143.
3. Cantey, J. R., Lushbaugh, W. B., and Inman, L. R. (1981): Attachment of bacteria to intestinal epithelial cells in diarrhea caused by *Escherichia coli* strain RDEC-1 in the rabbit: Stages and role of capsule. *J. Infect. Dis.*, 143:219–229.
4. Cravioto, A., Moyra, M., McConnell, B. et al. (1980): Studies of colonization factors in *Escherichia coli* strains isolated from humans: Identification and plesimed analysis. In: *Microbial Adhesion to Surface*, edited by R. C. W. Berkelay, pp. 530–532. Ellis Horwood, Sussex, England.
5. Gurwith, M. J., and Williams, T. W. (1977): Gastroenteritis in children: A two-year review in Manitoba. I. Etiology. *J. Infect. Dis.*, 136:239–247.
6. Kapikian, A. Z., Kim, H. W., Wyatt, R. G. et al. (1976): Human reovirus-like agent as the major pathogen associated with "winter" gastroenteritis in hospitalized infants and young children. *N. Engl. J. Med.*, 294:965–972.
7. Karunasagar, I. (1981): Production of remolysin by *Vibrio parahaemolyticus* in a chemically defined medium. *Appl. Environ. Microbiol.*, 41:1274–1275.

8. Karunasagar, I., Nagesha, C. N., and Bhat, J. V. (1979): Effect of metal ions on the production of vascular permeability factor by 569B strain of *Vibrio cholerae. Indian J. Med. Res.*, 69:18–25.

9. Konno, T., Suzuki, H., Inai, A. et al. (1978): A long term survey of rotavirus infection in Japanese children with acute gastroenteritis. *J. Infect. Dis.*, 138:569–576.

10. Pickering, L. K., Evans, Jr., D. J., Muñoz, O. et al. (1978): Prospective study of enteropathogens in children with diarrhea in Houston and Mexico. *J. Pediatr.*, 93:383–388.

11. Ruiz-Palacios, G. M., Escamilla, E., and Torres, J. (1982): Production of enterotoxins by *Campylobacter fetus* ssp *jejuni. 22nd Interscience Conference on Antimicrobial Agents and Chemotherapy*, Miami, Florida.

12. Ruiz-Palacios, G. M., Escamilla, E., and Torres, N. (1981): Experimental *Campylobacter* infection in chicken. *Infect. Immun.*, 34:250–255.

13. Shields, D. S., Kinehoff, L. V., Sauer, K. T., et al. (1982): Prospective studies of diarrhea illness in NE Brazil: Patterns of disease, etiologies and risk factors. *22nd Interscience Conference on Antimicrobial Agents and Chemotherapy*, Miami, Florida.

14. Ulshen, M. H., and Rollo, J. L. (1980): Pathogenesis of *Escherichia coli* gastroenteritis in man—another mechanism. *N. Engl. J. Med.*, 302:99–101.

15. Wood, L. V., Wolfe, W. H., Ruiz-Palacios, G. M. et al. (1982): An outbreak of gastroenteritis due to a heat-labile enterotoxin (LT)-producing strain of *Escherichia coli. 82nd Annual Meeting of the American Society for Microbiology*, Atlanta, Georgia.

Acute Diarrhea: Its Nutritional Consequences
in Children, edited by J. A. Bellanti.
Nestlé, Vevey/Raven Press, New York © 1983.

ETIOLOGIC AGENTS OF ACUTE DIARRHEA:
BACTERIAL AND PARASITIC

Discussion

Dr. Levine: Dr. Sack mentioned data in animals showing that strains that have lost their toxins but still contain adhesion colonization factor can cause diarrheal disease in neonatal animals. Also he raised the question as to whether that phenomenon is relevant or occurs in man. I would like to mention some instances where we think we have seen it occurring. We have had the opportunity in the past year or two to evaluate healthy volunteers and found in them two strains that lack toxins. One is a *Vibrio cholera* vaccine strain (Texas Star), and the other strain is an *Escherichia coli* that once was toxigenic and that lost its heat-labile and heat-stable toxins, but that still maintained colonization factor antigen 2 pili. Approximately 20% of individuals that were fed Texas Star strain had a very mild diarrheal response. We can show that this Texas Star strain colonizes rather avidly at the proximal end of the small intestine and does not revert to toxigenicity, suggesting that with that strain the diarrhea is apparently related to the colonization. With the nontoxigenic colonization factor antigen 2-positive strain, we have seen the same thing. Approximately 10% of individuals have mild diarrhea; one person had a mild to moderate diarrhea. We think this is an important observation because it may represent the price we will have to pay for attenuated strains against those pathogens, that is, acceptance of mild diarrhea in 20%, and maybe even moderate diarrhea in 1%.

With regard to Dr. Ruiz-Palacios's commentaries, we would like to corroborate and underline his statement that most toxigenic *E. coli* are still pathogens, and thus must have other adhesions. We think this is a very important point although not so long ago if it was suggested, one was considered an heretic. The sooner we accept this, the sooner we can attempt the development of vaccines that will give much broader spectrum protection.

Dr. Kapikian: Dr. Ruiz-Palacios, you mentioned that in the community in children under 2 years of age, 21% had enterotoxigenic *E. coli*, 18% rotavirus, and 15% *Campylobacter*; however, in patients hospitalized with gastroenteritis, rotavirus was present in about 50% of the cases. Could you put that into perspective for us? It would be helpful to underscore this point about severity of illness among these three agents. Where does the enterotoxigenic *E. coli* fit in hospitalizable gastroenteritis as compared with rotavirus?

Dr. Ruiz-Palacios: Yes, it is less frequent to find enterotoxigenic *E. coli* in patients who are admitted to the hospital. Two studies were conducted in Mexico, one in Mexico City where the prevalence was found to be 37%, and one conducted by the Social Security Service where the prevalence was found to be less than 4%.

Dr. Black: In the studies in Bangladesh, we were able to demonstrate that rotavirus was more commonly associated with dehydration; around 35% of episodes were associated with some detectable dehydration compared with 10 to 15% for *E. coli*, and a far lower percentage (2%) for all other types of diarrhea. This was in children less than 2 years of age in whom cholera was not found, with rare exceptions. In a similar way, at the treatment center, where we looked at the more severe cases of dehydration who probably had a good likelihood of dying without rehydration therapy, rotavirus was found in about 45% and *E. coli* in about 30%.

NUTRITIONAL CONSEQUENCES OF ACUTE
DIARRHEA IN CHILDREN

*Acute Diarrhea: Its Nutritional Consequences
in Children*, edited by J. A. Bellanti.
Nestlé, Vevey/Raven Press, New York © 1983.

Influence of Acute Diarrhea on the Growth Parameters of Children

*†Robert E. Black, *‡Kenneth H. Brown, and *Stan Becker

*International Centre for Diarrhoeal Diseases Research, Dacca, Bangladesh; †Center
for Vaccine Development, University of Maryland School of Medicine, Baltimore,
Maryland 21201; and ‡Division of Human Nutrition, Department of International
Health, Johns Hopkins University School of Hygiene and Public Health, Baltimore,
Maryland 21205

The physical growth of poor children in developing countries often falls far
below the standards of more affluent children in these countries, or of children
in developed countries. The growth of many children in developing countries
may be limited from reaching its full genetic potential by outside factors, such
as inadequate nutrient intake and morbidity from specific diseases.

The association between morbidity, especially the highly prevalent infectious
diseases, and malnutrition has been recognized for centuries; however, the
specific and quantitative relationships have been studied only in the past two
decades. From the early field studies done by Scrimshaw et al. and Mata et
al. in Guatemala came a more clear recognition of the importance of infectious
diseases, particularly diarrhea and measles, for their adverse effects on growth
(12,16). Later studies by Martorell in Guatemala were able to demonstrate
that children with frequent diarrhea had smaller weight and length increments
than children with less frequent diarrhea (11). Likewise, in The Gambia, Rowland et al. found a significant negative relationship between gastroenteritis and
weight and height gain (15). A similar negative relationship was found between
malaria and weight gain, but not for seven other categories of disease. Longitudinal studies in Mexico found that a high frequency of diarrhea, but not
of upper or lower respiratory infections, was associated with reduced weight
gain (6).

Although the importance of diarrheal diseases as frequent causes of illness
and as contributors to malnutrition has been well reported, the organisms
responsible for most of the diarrheal episodes could not be determined in
previous studies. However, in the past several years laboratory techniques have
become available to detect certain specific bacterial and viral agents that cause
diarrhea. It is now possible to identify an enteric pathogen in a majority of

episodes of diarrhea in young children. The use of these techniques in studies of the effects of diarrhea on growth should permit an evaluation of the anthropometic consequences of diarrheal illnesses associated with specific bacterial and viral pathogens.

To extend our understanding of the interactions between infectious diseases and the nutritional status of children, we initiated longitudinal studies in a cohort of young children in rural Bangladesh. We used a village-based surveillance system to determine the incidence, prevalence, and severity of malnutrition and a variety of diseases, including diarrhea associated with specific etiologic agents.

METHODS

The study was conducted in the Matlab Field Research area of the International Centre for Diarrhoeal Disease Research, Bangladesh. Two contiguous villages were selected and all children 2 to 48 months old in these villages were identified. Informed, signed consent was obtained for 177 (94%) of the available children. Twenty additional children born during the first year of study were added to the study when they were 2 months old (4).

A female field worker visited each child every other day to inquire about illness on that day or the preceding day. The field worker also examined the child for skin rashes, purulent discharge from nose or ears, or dehydration. A physician, who visited the child once per week, reviewed the information recorded by the field worker, obtained additional information, examined the child, and coded the presence or absence of specific illnesses on each day of the preceding week.

Illnesses were usually designated based on the physician's judgment; however, two illnesses had specific definitions. An upper respiratory illness was considered to be present if at least one of the following was noted: purulent nasal discharge, cough, or pharyngitis. An episode of diarrhea must have produced four or more liquid stools for at least 1 day, and that episode was considered resolved on any day with fewer than three stools. In this analysis of the first year of study, surveillance information on 61,536 days of observation is included.

On the first day that a child was noted to have diarrhea, two rectal swabs were obtained by the field worker. One swab was plated within several hours of collection, and agar plates were examined for enteric pathogens as previously described (3). From each stool, five lactose-positive *Escherichia coli*-like colonies and a pool of 10 similar colonies were tested for heat-labile toxin (LT) by the Chinese hamster ovary cell assay and for heat-stable toxin (ST) by the infant mouse assay. Fecal material from the other swab was tested for rotavirus by an enzyme-linked immunosorbent assay (ELISA).

Anthropometric indicators were measured on the first 2 days of each calendar month, or in the next week if a child was away from home on the day of measurement (5). Nude or lightly clothed children were weighed to the nearest 0.1 kg on a spring scale (Salter) and recumbent length was measured to the nearest 0.1 cm on a wooden platform with a sliding footboard. Mid-upper-arm circumference and triceps skinfold thickness were measured as previously described.

The children's measurements were used to establish reference curves for growth patterns present in the study villages (5). The smoothed curves were fitted using linear and higher-order polynomial regression analysis. These internal reference standards enabled age-independent comparisons of all children within the study population by relating their actual anthropometric status to the village norms (1,5). The actual anthropometric measurements were also compared with appropriate external reference populations and these results reported previously (1,5).

For analysis of the relationship between infectious diseases and growth in various time periods, we used the proportion of days in that period that a given illness was present as an independent variable for that child. Depending on the specific analysis, we used a variety of measures of physical growth. At times, we used actual weights and lengths, or changes in these between two assessments. For other analyses, we compared the child's measurements with the village reference curves and expressed his or her weight or length as a percentage of that expected for a child of that age and sex, or his or her growth rate as a percentage of that expected based on the village reference curves. Statistical methods included analysis of variance, linear regression, and step-wise multiple regression (most significant first).

RESULTS

The fitted curves of weight by age indicated that at 6 months of age, village children averaged only 79% of the external reference population (National Center for Health Statistics, NCHS) median children. Village children gained weight with increasing age; however, their nutritional status, expressed as a percentage of the NCHS median, continued to decline until 14 to 17 months of age. Girls were smaller than boys, both by absolute criteria and relative to external reference children of the same age.

According to the fitted curves for length by age, village children averaged 85 to 90% of the NCHS median length. Village boys and girls were initially stunted to a similar degree, but girls became even shorter relative to the NCHS population with increasing age.

By prospective surveillance, an illness was noted on 75% of all days of observation. Upper respiratory illnesses were found on 60% of all days. Diarrhea was present on 13% of days, and skin infections were also quite prevalent. During the first year of study, 941 episodes of diarrhea were identified, and 920 of these were studied for enteric pathogens. A pathogen was found in 51% of these episodes, with enterotoxigenic *E. coli* accounting for 27% of episodes as a single infection and 4% in combination with another pathogen (Table 1). Shigellae were the second most frequent pathogens, and rotaviruses third.

The incidence of all diarrhea was highest in the first year of life and declined progressively with age from 7 to 4 episodes per child per year (Fig. 1). *E. coli* diarrhea annual incidence decreased from two episodes per child in the youngest age group to one episode in older children. Rotavirus diarrhea incidence was about one-half an episode per year per child for the first 2 years of life. *Shigella*-associated diarrhea had a peak incidence in children in the third year of life.

The median duration of the various types of diarrhea was 4 to 5 days except shigellosis, which had a duration of 7 days (Table 2). With all types of diarrhea, a substantial proportion of episodes persisted for 10 days or more; however, the proportion of long episodes was higher for diarrhea associated with *Shigella* or *E. coli* than with rotavirus.

In assessing the impact of diarrhea on growth, we first examined the effect of acute episodes of specific types of diarrhea on the weights of young children. Since study children were being weighed each month, weights for the 2 months preceding the acute episode were available for most children. After diarrhea was identified by surveillance workers, return home visits were made and children were weighed on the second and fourth days of illness (in a few cases the diarrhea resolved after 3 days but the fourth day weight was still obtained to permit the inclusion of these children in the analysis). Diarrheal episodes were selected for analyses if either rotavirus or enterotoxigenic *E. coli* were found in the stool, if the child was 6 to 24 months of age (average 15 and 16 months for *E. coli* and rotavirus groups, respectively), if the illness lasted less than 7 days (median 4 days), if no other serious illnesses occurred within 4 weeks after diarrhea, and if all weight measurements before, during, and after

TABLE 1. *Enteropathogens identified during diarrhea in a cohort of 197 children*[a]

Enteropathogen	Number	Percentage
Enterotoxigenic *Escherichia coli*	248	27.0
Shigella	118	12.8
Rotavirus	35	3.8
E. coli and *Shigella*	26	2.8
Non-O group 1 *Vibrio*	10	1.1
E. coli and rotavirus	6	0.7
Giardia lamblia	5	0.5
Vibrio cholerae O group 1	3	0.3
Shigella and rotavirus	2	0.2
Entamoeba histolytica	2	0.2
Other	10	1.1
None	455	49.5
Total	920	100.0

[a] Children aged 2 to 60 months.

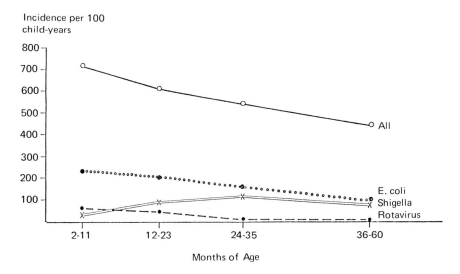

FIG. 1. Annual incidence of diarrhea by enteropathogen and age in a cohort of children in rural Bangladesh.

illness were obtained. None of the episodes were associated with clinically detectable dehydration and all were treated with kaolin.

Children during either *E. coli* or rotavirus diarrhea weighed 250 to 350 g less than they had at the last routine weighing (average of 2 weeks before the episode). Some of the weight loss may have been due to temporary fluid deficits from diarrheal losses; however, 1 week after recovery from diarrhea, the children still weighed less than they had at the prior weighing. Children did not recover their prior weight until 2 weeks after diarrhea. Moreover, in spite of some catch-up growth between 1 and 4 weeks postdiarrhea, children's weights remained slightly below the weight that would have been expected if these children had continued the rate of growth that they had prior to their illness.

TABLE 2. *Duration of diarrheal episodes[a] associated with enterotoxigenic Escherichia coli, Shigella, or rotavirus, and of episodes without an identified enteropathogen*

Enteropathogen	Total episodes	Duration (days)				
		% Distribution				
		1–3	4–9	10–19	≥ 20	Median
Escherichia coli	248	44	32	17	7	5
Shigella	118	23	39	21	16	7
Rotavirus	35	43	37	17	3	4
None	455	31	44	17	8	5

[a] Excludes episodes with isolation of multiple pathogens.

The patterns of weight loss and gain were similar for rotavirus and *E. coli* diarrhea.

To evaluate the relative importance of the prevalent infectious diseases as causes of growth faltering, we compared the growth rates of children in 60-day periods as a function of the proportion of days in that period that specific illnesses were present. Growth rates for each 2-month period were expressed as a percentage of the weight or length growth rate for an average child of that age in the study villages. Periods with higher proportions of days with upper respiratory or skin infections did not have significantly poorer weight or length growth rates. In contrast, periods with higher proportions of days with diarrhea had lower weight gain rates ($p = 0.02$) (Fig. 2). Periods with more days of diarrhea associated with enterotoxigenic *E. coli* also had poorer weight growth rates ($p = 0.04$). Periods with rotavirus- or *Shigella*-associated diarrhea did not have significantly lower weight gain rates; however, periods with *more Shigella*-associated diarrhea had diminished length growth rates ($p = 0.008$) (Fig. 3). Periods with any diarrhea, or with *E. coli* or rotavirus diarrhea, did not have significantly lower length growth rates.

The relationship between the proportion of days in 60-day periods with illnesses and growth was also assessed by stepwise multiple regression analysis using change in weight status (expressed as a percentage of the village reference standard for age) as the dependent variable. When the independent variables included the initial weight and the proportions of days in the period with upper respiratory, skin, or diarrheal infections, only initial weight and diarrhea had significant negative regression coefficients. The multiple r was 0.15. When the independent variables included the initial weight, and the proportions of the period ill with diarrhea associated with *E. coli*, *Shigella*, or rotavirus, or with

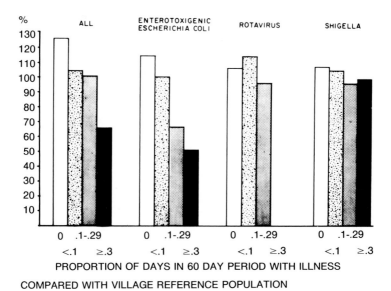

FIG. 2. Average percentage of expected bimonthly weight gain rate by proportion of days with selected types of diarrhea during 60-day periods.

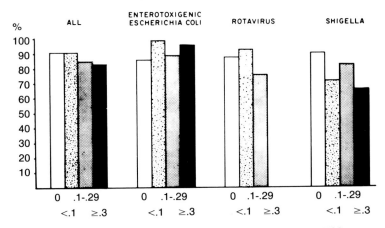

PROPORTION OF DAYS IN 60 DAY PERIOD WITH ILLNESS

COMPARED WITH VILLAGE REFERENCE POPULATION

FIG. 3. Average percentage of expected bimonthly length increase rate by proportion of days with selected types of diarrhea during 60-day periods.

no detectable pathogen, only initial weight and *E. coli* diarrhea entered the regression with significant negative coefficients (multiple $r = 0.132$).

We also performed linear regressions of change in length status on proportion of days with selected common illnesses in one year periods (Table 3). Diarrhea was the only common illness variable with a significant coefficient. Furthermore, diarrhea associated with *Shigella*, *E. coli*, or not associated with a recognized pathogen, had significantly different regression coefficients.

TABLE 3. *Coefficients and levels of significance for regressions of change in length status in one year on proportion of days with selected illnesses*

	Dependent variable of regression	
	Change in length status (% of village reference for age)	
Independent variable[a]	Coefficient	*p* Value
Upper respiratory illness	—	NS[b]
Skin infection	—	NS
Diarrhea	−0.038	0.008
Shigella diarrhea	−0.081	0.026
Escherichia coli diarrhea	−0.060	0.045
"No pathogen" diarrhea	−0.046	0.049
Rotavirus diarrhea	—	NS

[a] Initial length entered into regression before test variables.

[b] Not significant ($p > 0.05$).

To investigate the relative impact of the different types of diarrhea on change in length status in a 1-year period, we used a stepwise multiple regression analysis. Only *Shigella* diarrhea had a significant negative coefficient, and the other types of diarrhea did not add to the regression (multiple $r = 0.173$).

DISCUSSION

Children with diarrhea often lose weight, possibly due to associated catabolism, decreased food intake, and/or malabsorption of nutrients. Children with selected, relatively mild, enterotoxigenic *E. coli* or rotavirus diarrheal illnesses did not regain the lost weight until nearly 2 weeks after the illness. In spite of some catch-up growth during the convalescent period while eating their usual diet, the children did not approach their expected weight level until 4 weeks after illness. It could be anticipated that the nutritional consequences of such an illness would be worse if sufficient food were not available to permit even the limited catch-up growth. Furthermore, it is likely that weight loss or stagnation would be more severe with diarrheal episodes of longer duration. It is also clear that the occurrence of another serious illness during convalescence from diarrhea could prevent catch-up growth and result in further weight loss.

In these studies, diarrhea was the only illness that had a consistent and significant adverse effect on growth. Diarrhea prevalence had an inverse relationship with the change in weight status in 2-month periods and on the change in length status over 1 year.

Diarrhea due to enterotoxigenic *E. coli* was the only specific type of diarrhea that had a significant negative effect on the bimonthly weight growth of children in this community, and diarrhea with *Shigella* had the strongest negative effect on annual length growth. Although the prevalence of a type of diarrhea must have some importance in determining the magnitude of the nutritional losses to a community, the high prevalence of these two types of diarrhea is probably not the only explanation, since diarrhea for which a pathogen could not be found accounted for one-half of all diarrheal episodes and was not associated with growth faltering.

With both *E. coli* and *Shigella* diarrheas, a sizable number of episodes lasted more than 10 or even 20 days, and it was these episodes that had the most profound effect on growth. *E. coli* diarrhea is usually self-limited with a duration of less than 1 week, even in cases with extensive fluid loss (13). The reason for the long duration of some *E. coli* illnesses is unknown; however, one possible explanation could be that the initial small bowel infection leads to a malabsorption syndrome which, in turn, prolongs the diarrhea. The explanation for the episodes of long duration with *Shigella* infections may be different. *Shigella* is a pathogen that invades the colon, and severe disease is often associated with a long duration of dysentery (7,8). Chronic diarrhea, associated with deep ulcerations in the colon, has been noted to follow the acute illness in a small percentage of persons with shigellosis and is said to be more common in poorly nourished children (7–9,14). Both acute and prolonged episodes of dysentery may result in extensive loss of blood (and serum proteins) from the colonic ulcerations. Thus, in addition to the effects of diarrhea on catabolism, decreased food intake, and malabsorption, shigellosis results in loss of protein which, for children on a marginal diet, must be compensated by increased dietary intake for optimal growth to occur. Children in this study were demonstrated to have usual dietary protein intakes that were less than 90% of the recommended safe level of intake (2). The fecal loss of protein was probably not compensated by higher dietary intake and may have been partially responsible for growth faltering in children with shigellosis. The particular effect of shigellosis in limiting linear growth is also consistent with previous observations that protein intake was an important determinant of length (10).

These analyses are not merely of academic interest. A better understanding of the frequency of specific illnesses and of the determinants of malnutrition in children of developing countries should permit more rational design of health and nutrition interventions. From these analyses, we could predict that control of diarrhea due to enterotoxigenic *E. coli* and *Shigella* would reduce diarrhea morbidity by 40%, improve the growth of young children, and reduce malnutrition.

REFERENCES

1. Brown, K. H., Black, R. E., and Becker, S. (1982): Seasonal changes in nutritional status and the prevalence of malnutrition in a longitudinal study of young children in rural Bangladesh. *Am. J. Clin. Nutr.*, 36:303–313.
2. Brown, K. H., Black, R. E., Becker, S., Nahar, S., and Sawyer, J. (1982): Consumption of foods and nutrients by weanlings in rural Bangladesh. *Am. J. Clin. Nutr.*, 36:878–889.
3. Black, R. E., Brown, K. H., Becker, S., Alim, A. R. M. A., and Huq, I. (1982): Longitudinal studies of infection and physical growth of children in rural Bangladesh. II. Incidence of diarrhea and association with known pathogens. *Am. J. Epidemiol.*, 115:315–324.
4. Black, R. E., Brown, K. H., Becker, S., and Yunus, M. (1982): Longitudinal studies of infectious diseases and physical growth of children in rural Bangladesh. I. Patterns of morbidity. *Am. J. Epidemiol.*, 115:305–314.
5. Brown, K. H., Black, R. E., Becker, S. and Hoque, A. (1982): Patterns of physical growth in a longitudinal study of young children in rural Bangladesh. *Am. J. Clin. Nutr.*, 36:294–302.
6. Condon-Paoloni, D., Cravioto, J., Johnston, F. E., de Licardie, E. R., and O'Scholl, T. (1977): Morbidity and growth of infants and young children in a rural Mexican village. *Am. J. Public Health*, 67:651–656.
7. Davison, W. C. (1922): A bacteriologic and clinical consideration of bacillary dysentery in adults and children. *Medicine*, 1:389–510.
8. Felsen, J. (1945): *Bacillary Dysentery Colitis and Enteritis*, pp. 290–464. Saunders, Philadelphia.
9. Fletcher, W. C., and MacKinnon, D. L. (1919): A contribution to the study of chronicity in dysentery carriers. *Med. Res. Counc. Spec. Rep. Ser. (Lond.)*, 29:14–19.
10. Graham, G. G., Creed, H. M., MacLean, W. C., Jr. et al. (1981): Determinants of growth among poor children: nutrient intake—achieved growth relationships. *Am. J. Clin. Nutr.*, 34:539–554.
11. Martorell, R., Habicht, J.-P., Yarbrough, C., Lechtig, A., Klein, R. E., and Western, K. A. (1975): Acute morbidity and physical growth in rural Guatemalan children. *Am. J. Dis. Child.*, 129:1296–1301.

12. Mata, L. J., Kromal, R. A., Urrutia, J. J., and Garcia, B. (1977): Effect of infection on food intake and the nutritional state: perspectives as viewed from the village. *Am. J. Clin. Nutr.,* 30:1215–1227.

13. Merson, M. H., and Black, R. E. (1981): Enterotoxigenic Escherichia coli diarrhea. In: *Acute Enteric Infections in Children. New Prospects for Treatment and Prevention,* pp 81–92. Elsevier/North-Holland, Amsterdam.

14. Perry, H. M. (1925): Laboratory research on ancillary dysentery. *J. R. Army Med. Corps,* 45:345–349.

15. Rowland, M. G. M., Cole, T. J., and Whitehead, R. G. (1977): A quantitative study into the role of infection in determining nutritional status in Gambian village children. *Br. J. Nutr.,* 37:441–450.

16. Scrimshaw, N. S. (1970): Synergism of malnutrition and infection: evidence from field studies in Guatemala. *JAMA,* 212:1685–1692.

Acute Diarrhea: Its Nutritional Consequences in Children, edited by J. A. Bellanti.
Nestlé, Vevey/Raven Press, New York © 1983.

INFLUENCE ON THE GROWTH
PARAMETERS OF CHILDREN

Comments

Leonardo Mata

*Instituto de Investigaciones en Salud (INISA), Universidad de Costa Rica,
Ciudad Universitaria Rodrigo Facio, San Pedro, Costa Rica*

Microorganisms have played a prominent role in the evolutionary development of the gastrointestinal tract of vertebrates. Through eons, the human intestinal mucosa has evolved in intimate association with myriads of bacteria, and with viruses and parasites, to such an extent that the majority of microbial species are "indigenous" or "autochthonous" to the human host (10). There are several microbial habitats in the intestinal milieu (Fig. 1); the lumen and interplical spaces (virtual or filled with pabulum) apparently are of similar nature, unless proof of existing difference is contributed (17). Plicae and villi are much more numerous in the duodenum, jejunum, and proximal ileum than in the terminal ileum and colon. It may be necessary for pathogens to reach beyond these spaces to cause harm; those reaching intervilli spaces have greater opportunities for attachment and for invasion of the mucosa. Intervillous spaces provide a different habitat in that biochemical cell activity, secretion by goblet cells, and extrusion of cells and nutrients are prominent in this area. In malnutrition, chronic malabsorption, or other pathologic processes, there is formation of hollow spaces or microcaverns (17), possibly permitting stagnation of secretions and cell debris. Bacteria associate with crypt cells and they dwell deep in the crypt. Bacteria and other agents adhere to villi epithelium, usually at the tips. Agents may be loosely associated, but pathogens are more intimately so. *Cryptosporidium* attaches to the microvilli border of enterocytes, forms a basilar plate and disturbs the brush border; it may locate under the microcalyx (31). *Giardia* adheres firmly to the mucosal surface and causes anatomical and functional alterations associated with malabsorption (11). Other agents invade epithelial cells and replicate within them, causing profound structural damage, as do rotaviruses (8). Other agents such as *Shigella* invade the epithelial cell to burrow into the lamina propria, where they cause an inflammatory response with abscess formation and eventual mucosal ulceration (13). Finally, other organisms actually translocate to reach the lymph and blood circulation, to home in distant organs, such as occurs with salmonellosis (29).

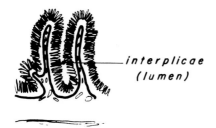

interplicae
(lumen)

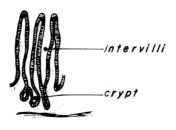

intervilli

crypt

FIG. 1. Schematic representation of different habitats in the intestinal lumen of man. While toxin-producing bacteria may induce pathogenic actions from the interplicae spaces, most agents initiate their pathogenesis after adhering to the surface of the enterocyte, or by penetrating and multiplying in this cell. Some agents invade the lamina propria and still others translocate this barrier to reach the lymph and blood circulation. (After ref. 17.)

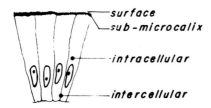

surface
sub-microcalix

intracellular

intercellular

It is then easy to accept that the close interactions between pathogen and host will be translated in important physiological and nutritional alterations.

NUTRITIONAL IMPACT

The negative nutritional effects of diarrhea result from reduced food consumption, reduced nutrient absorption, increased secretion, protein-losing enteropathy, and metabolic alterations.

Reduced Food Consumption

Diarrhea interferes with proper consumption of the usual diet. Such an effect is due to one or more of the following symptoms and signs: anorexia, vomiting, dehydration, fever, discomfort, and anxiety. Furthermore, cultural traditions and beliefs often result in parental suppression of food for days or weeks after an attack of diarrhea (30). Prospective observations in cohorts of

TABLE 1. *Clinical features of specific infectious diarrhea in children observed from birth to 2 years (Puriscal, Costa Rica, 1979–1981)*

Diarrhea	No. of episodes	Number (%) with				
		Anorexia	Fever	Vomiting	Dehydration	Fecal blood
Rotavirus	43	15 (35)	22 (51)	18 (42)	4 (9)	0
Campylobacter	17	8 (47)	7 (41)	6 (35)	0	4 (23)
Shigella	6	3 (50)	3 (50)	0	0	5 (83)
Total	66	26 (39)	32 (48)	24 (36)	4 (6)	9 (14)

Guatemalan and Costa Rican rural children living under varying environmental conditions (21,22) revealed that anorexia and vomiting are common findings of diarrhea (Table 1). The immediate consequence of such symptoms is mild to severe restriction of food intake for days or weeks. Prospective weekly dietary surveys in weaned children showed that as much as 20 to 50% of the total home diet is not consumed due to diarrhea alone (Table 2; ref. 20). Further evidence for reduced food consumption in diarrheas was obtained in Uganda (34) and Bangladesh (25). The Bengali workers also demonstrated that the effect diminished 2 weeks after recuperation, but was not totally corrected then, especially in rotavirus and enterotoxigenic *Escherichia coli* (ETEC) diarrhea (Table 3). This study is particularly relevant to developing countries, as it strengthens observations made in Guatemala (23) that village children who have suffered from malnutrition consume adequate quantities of nutrients during healthy periods, while the presence of diarrhea impairs consumption and absorption of macronutrients, an effect persisting for several weeks after the episode.

TABLE 2. *Mean daily food consumption during acute diarrheal disease in Guatemalan and Ugandan children*

Age (months)	Guatemala[a]				Uganda[b]	
	Protein (g)		Energy (MJ)		Energy (MJ)	
	Well	Diarrhea	Well	Diarrhea	Well	Diarrhea
25–30	25	19	3.82	3.02	3.52	1.89
31–36					3.95	2.03
% Change well-diarrhea	24		21		48	

[a] Unpublished data.
[b] After ref. 34.

TABLE 3. *Energy intake during and after occurrence of specific diarrheal disease in preschool children in Bangladesh[a]*

Diarrhea	Acute phase	Recovery	
		2 weeks	8 weeks
Rotavirus	68.5 ± 22.6	87.2 ± 26.2	115.0 ± 20.2
Shigella	70.0 ± 28.2	100.5 ± 27.8	109.3 ± 18.8
Cholera	74.9 ± 36.2	111.1 ± 35.4	109.6 ± 31.7
ETEC	70.7 ± 37.9	91.0 ± 28.4	114.9 ± 19.0

[a] Energy intake in kcal/kg/day. Mean ± SD.
Adapted from ref. 25.

Reduced Absorption of Nutrients

Adhesion of bacteria to the mucosa, release of toxins, direct damage to the enterocyte and crypt cells, bacterial hydrolysis of bile acids and carbohydrates, and other pathogenic actions result in a diminished capacity of the mucosa to absorb macro- and micronutrients (12,14,15,16). The Bengali workers recently showed a decreased absorption of nitrogen, calories, fat, and carbohydrate in children with specific diarrheas; the effect was apparently, but not totally, corrected 8 weeks after termination of diarrhea (Table 4; ref. 26).

Increased Secretion

Diarrhea is a state of hypersecretion. In rotavirus infection, there is a clear movement of water from the infected segment of the small intestine into the lumen, resulting in a decreased sodium flux from the lumen to the extracellular fluid (ECF) and an increased sodium flux from the ECF into the lumen (15). These alterations are related to damage and lysis of villous tips with replace-

TABLE 4. *Coefficient of absorption during and after occurrence of specific diarrheal disease in preschool children in Bangladesh[a]*

Diarrhea	Nutrient	Acute phase	Recovery	
			2 weeks	8 weeks
Rotavirus	Nitrogen	43.3 ± 22.3	68.5 ± 13.0	59.9 ± 28.2
	Calories	54.4 ± 23.7	91.1 ± 4.6	81.2 ± 10.1
Shigella	Nitrogen	41.3 ± 45.6	73.6 ± 4.8	72.3 ± 9.7
	Calories	68.1 ± 32.0	79.7 ± 13.9	90.4 ± 2.5
ETEC	Nitrogen	58.3 ± 13.9	54.0 ± 33.3	72.8 ± 9.3
	Calories	86.7 ± 7.7	82.2 ± 10.9	88.7 ± 6.5

[a] Coefficient of absorption per kg per day, mean ± SD.
Adapted from ref. 25.

TABLE 5. *Effects of enteric infection on intestinal secretion*

Action	Effect
Imbalance of digestive-absorptive processes	
Hydrostatic pressure by vascular obstruction and epithelial cell loss	Loss of fluid, electrolytes, fat and protein
Cyclic AMP and cyclic GMP stimulation by enterotoxins, bile and fatty acids, hormones, neurotransmitters	Active secretion of water and electrolytes
Greater calcium cell permeability induced by mediators	

ment of absorptive enterocytes by immature crypt-like cells. There is no alteration of cyclic adenosine monophosphate (AMP) concentrations.

Other causes of hypersecretion are stimulation of cyclic AMP and cyclic guanosine monophosphate (GMP) by heat-labile toxins and heat-stable toxins released by enteric bacteria, or by increased concentrations of bile and fatty acids from bacterial metabolism, or by hormones and neurotransmitters (Table 5; ref. 12). Other possible causes are listed in Table 5. The hypersecretory state results in important deficits in sodium, potassium, chloride, and water (18), and probably in many other elements such as vitamins and trace elements.

Nutrient Losses

Similar to the measles-induced abrupt fall in plasma albumin through a protein-losing enteropathy (9), structural alterations in the mucosal epithelium with *Shigella*, rotaviruses, and probably *Campylobacter*, result in a "protein-losing enteropathy." An increased ratio of α_1-antitrypsin (stool over serum concentrations) was observed in about half of rotavirus diarrheas and even more frequently in shigellosis (Table 6; ref. 33). The alteration consists of losses

TABLE 6. *Ratio of α_1-antitrypsin (stool/serum) in specific diarrheal disease in Bangladeshi children and adults*

Diarrhea	No. of patients	α_1-AT ratio			
		< 1	1–2	3+	Total 1+
Shigella	15	2	9	4	13 (87)[a]
ETEC	11	4	6	1	7 (64)
Rotavirus	14	8	6	0	6 (43)

[a] Relative percentage in parentheses.

of plasma and epithelial and blood cells, particularly when there is tissue in-
volvement, as in shigellosis. The consequences for malnourished children
might be more serious, because in chronic malnutrition there is already a
marked thinning of the intestinal wall (7). The protein-losing enteropathy
seems to be an explanation for the occurrence of outbreaks of kwashiorkor
a few weeks after epidemics of diarrhea.

Other Metabolic Alterations

Acute diarrhea leads to malnutrition, which becomes worse if prompt rehydration and alimentation are not instituted. Metabolic alterations such as
those described in systemic infections (2) are to be expected. Negative balances
of nitrogen, magnesium, potassium, and phosphorus; mobilization of amino
acids from muscle for gluconeogenesis; augmented synthesis of acute-phase
reactant proteins; and sequestration of trace elements are important phenomena that are likely to occur in all diarrheas.

GROWTH AND DEVELOPMENT IMPACT

Diarrhea induces acute weight loss and arrest in linear growth, as other
infections do. Detailed observation of this phenomenon was possible through
prospective studies of village children in their natural ecosystems in Guatemala
and Costa Rica (21,22). Inspection of individual growth curves of 45 cohort
children showed a consistent pattern of relative absence of diarrhea during
exclusive breast-feeding; the nutritional status of infants was noted to be adequate, even if they had experienced fetal growth retardation or had been born
prematurely. With the onset of weaning (a protracted process starting at about
3 months of life and continuing throughout the second year of life) a variety
of infections associated with faltering of the weight and height curves was
recorded in each child. Previous description of 20 growth histories selected
among the 45 cohort children revealed a consistent pattern of progressive
weight deterioration (wastage) with infections. Figure 2 illustrates the intestinal
infections and body length during the first 2 years of life for a Guatemalan
child born with adequate birth weight and length, in comparison with the 50th
percentile of the National Center for Health Statistics reference curve (27). An
etiologic association was defined as the occurrence of a pathogen 1 week before
or after onset of a diarrheal episode. Four of the nine diarrheal episodes were
related to one or more pathogens (22). Five diarrheas were not associated with
agents; *Campylobacter* and ETEC were not investigated at the time of the
study (1964–1969). Diarrhea was related to periods of faltering and the sum-
mation of all such events ended in marked growth retardation (stunting), already evident by 1 year of age. The stunting effect was more marked if the
child had experienced fetal growth retardation, a common event in Guatemalan Indian villages (21). In addition to the stunting effect, there was weight
loss or failure to thrive, which eventually resulted in wastage.

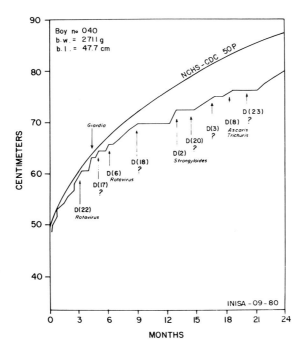

FIG. 2. Body length curve, diarrhea episodes, and enteric pathogenic agents in a child from the Cauqué Study born with an adequate weight for gestational age. Comparison is made with the 50th percentile of the NCHS growth curve. Although the child was breast-fed, diarrhea occurred particularly after weaning began. Often enteric agents were associated with the diarrhea. Most diarrhea episodes were associated with periods of stunting. (After ref. 22.)

It can be concluded that diarrheas are a major cause of chronic malnutrition (wastage) and stunting of village children, especially when there is fetal growth retardation. A negative effect of diarrhea on growth has been described in several studies (3,6,19). Wasted and/or stunted children, on the other hand, are more prone to suffer from a more severe course of diarrhea and also exhibit a higher risk of death, as evidenced in field studies in Guatemala, India, Bangladesh, and the Gambia (e.g., see refs. 5 and 21).

OTHER PUBLIC HEALTH IMPACTS

Morbidity

A long-term prospective study in Guatemala (21) revealed about eight episodes of diarrhea per child per year; surveillance every 2 weeks yields a lower figure (1). Projection of these figures to Latin America gives about 100 million cases of diarrhea for 1976 using the low estimate, or 350 million cases if it is assumed that each child experiences seven episodes per year (21,24). Since rotaviruses are associated with greater dehydration than other agents (32,35), their contribution to chronic malnutrition and to precipitation of marasmus and kwashiorkor must be considerable.

Mortality

Mortality due to diarrhea is exceedingly high in Latin America as contrasted with North America. An assumed lethality of 1 per 1,000 cases would give about 100,000 deaths under 5 years of age in Latin America in 1976, which is close to the reported figure of 94,077 deaths (28). This could be an underestimate as lethality may be greater, especially in rural areas where there is no provision for rehydration. Lethality of rotavirus diarrhea seems lower than that due to *Shigella* and *Salmonella* (4). However, the marked dehydration in rotavirus diarrhea observed in Guatemala and Costa Rica (32,35) suggests the seriousness of rotavirus diarrhea. Autopsy studies are needed to assess the contribution of each etiology to diarrheal death. The risk of death increases in malnourished children (Table 7; ref. 5). Thus, diarrhea is a malnourishing factor, and malnutrition enhances risk of death, a dreadful vicious circle.

COMMENT

Field studies revealed that children suffer from two to eight diarrhea episodes per person per year during the first 3 years of life, equivalent to an estimated 100 million diarrhea cases in children under 5 years of age in 1976 in Latin America; this represents too much wasting, stunting, and suffering.

Diarrhea is often accompanied by anorexia, which limits food consumption by village children already consuming a deficient diet. Several functional al-

TABLE 7. *Mortality rate after anthropometric assessment in Bangladesh, 1975–1976*

Nutritional status (% Harvard values)	No. of children	Deaths per 1,000 children	
		0–11[a]	12–23[a]
Weight/height			
> 90	399	35.1	17.5
80–89	979	26.6	26.6
70–79	566	28.3	21.2
< 70	75	66.7	80.0
Height/age			
> 95	182	16.5	16.5
90–94	656	22.9	16.8
85–89	713	28.0	9.8
< 85	468	51.3	62.0

[a] Months after anthropometric assessment.
Adapted from ref. 5.

terations result in malabsorption; a protein-losing enteropathy attributed to loss of plasma and cells has been described. Diarrhea induces wasting and stunting, more evident in small-for-gestational-age infants, or in children deprived of human milk, or in those living under adverse environmental conditions. Diarrhea is an important cause of wastage, stunting, and severe malnutrition.

If severe dehydration is not promptly corrected, death ensues. The death toll for Latin America was about 100,000 in 1976. This point alone justifies all efforts for provision of primary health services, including oral rehydration programs, promotion of breast-feeding, and adequate alimentation during the first 2 years of life. It also justifies research on the mechanisms of disease transmission, and on alternate avenues of control and prevention.

REFERENCES

1. Barua, D. (1981): In: *Acute Enteric Infections in Children. New Prospects for Treatment and Prevention*, edited by T. Holme, J. Holmgren, M. H. Merson, and R. Mollby, pp. 1–6. Elsevier/North-Holland, Amsterdam.
2. Beisel, W. R. (1977): *Am. J. Clin. Nutr.*, 30:1236–1247.
3. Black, R. E., Brown, K. H., and Becker, S. (1982): *International Conference on Acute Diarrhea in Children: Nutritional Implications*, Washington, D.C.
4. Black, R. E., Merson, M. H., Rahman, A. S. M. M., Yanus, M., Alim, A. R. M. A., Hug, I., Yolken, R. H., and Curlin, G. T. (1980): *J. Infect. Dis.*, 142:660–664.
5. Chen, L., Alauddin-Chowdhury, A. K. M., and Huffman, S. L. (1980): *Am. J. Clin. Nutr.*, 33:1836–1845.
6. Cole, T. J., and Parkin, J. M. (1977): *Trans. Roy. Soc. Trop. Med. Hyg.*, 71:196–198.
7. Cramer, B. (1964): *Br. Med. J.*, 2:1373–1375.
8. Davidson, G. P., and Barnes, G. L. (1979): *Acta Paediatr. Scand.*, 68:181–186.
9. Doseter, J. F. B., and Whittle, H. C. (1975): *Br. Med. J.*, 2:592–593.
10. Dubos, R., Schaedler, R. W., Costella, R., and Hoet, P. (1965): *J. Exp. Med.*, 122:67–72.
11. Erlandsen, S. L., and Chase, D. G. (1974): *Am. J. Clin. Nutr.*, 27:1277–1286.
12. Field, M. (1978): In: *Etiology, Pathophysiology, and Treatment of Acute Gastroenteritis*, pp. 57–61. Seventy-Fourth Ross Conference Pediatric Research, Columbus, Ohio.
13. Formal, S. B., Abrams, C. D., Schneider, H., and Spring, H. (1963): *J. Bacteriol.*, 85:119–125.
14. Guerrant, R. L. (1983): *Rev. Infect. Dis.* (in press).
15. Hamilton, J. R., Gall, D. G., Butler, D. G., and Middleton, P. J. (1976): In: *Acute Diarrhoea in Childhood*. Ciba Foundation Symposium No. 42 (new series), pp. 209–219. Elsevier, Excerpta Medica, North-Holland, Amsterdam.
16. Keusch, G. T. (1983): *Rev. Infect. Dis.* (in press).
17. Luckey, T. D. (1974): *Am. J. Clin. Nutr.*, 27:1266–1276.
18. Mahalanabis, D. (1981): In: *Acute Enteric Infections in Children. New Prospects for Treatment and Prevention*, edited by T. Holme, J. Holmgren, M. H. Merson, and R. Mollby, pp. 303–318. Elsevier/North-Holland, Amsterdam.
19. Martorell, R., Habicht, J. P., Yarbrough, C. et al. (1975): *Am. J. Dis. Child.*, 129:1296–1301.
20. Mata, L. (1979): *Proc. Nutr. Soc.*, 38:29–40.
21. Mata, L. J. (1978): *The Children of Santa María Cauqué. A Prospective Field Study of Health and Growth*. MIT Press, Cambridge, Massachusetts.
22. Mata, L., Jiménez, P., Allen, M. A., Vargas, W., García, M. E., Urrutia, J. J., and Wyatt, R. G. (1981): In: *Acute Enteric Infections in Children. New Prospects for Treatment and Prevention*, edited by T. Holme, J. Holmgren, M. H. Merson, and R. Mollby, pp. 233–251. Elsevier/North-Holland, Amsterdam.
23. Mata, L. J., Kronmal, R. A., Urrutia, J. J., and Gacia, B. (1977): *Am. J. Clin. Nutr.*, 30:1215–1227.

24. Mata, L., Kronmal, R. A., and Villegas, H. (1980): In: *Cholera and Related Diarrheas: Molecular Aspects of a Global Health Problem*, edited by O. Ouchterlony and J. Holmgren, pp. 1–14. S. Karger, Basel.
25. Molla, A. M., Molla, A., Sarker, S. A., and Rahaman, M. M. (1981): *ICDDR, B.*, Dacca, Bangladesh. Working Paper No. 20.
26. Molla, A., Molla, A. M., Sarker, S. A., Khatoon, M., and Rahaman, M. M. (1981): *ICDDR, B.*, Dacca, Bangladesh. Working Paper No. 19.
27. National Center for Health Statistics (NCHS) (1974): *NCHS Growth Curves for Children. Birth to 18 Years.* U.S. DHEW Pub. No. (PHS) 78-1650. U.S. Department of Health, Education and Welfare, Public Health Service, Hyattsville, Maryland.
28. Oficina Panamericana de la Salud (PAHO-O.P.S.) (1980): *Bol. Epidemiol.*, 1:1–4.
29. Saphra, J., and Winter, J. W. (1957): *N. Engl. J. Med.*, 256:1128–1134.
30. Scrimshaw, N. S., Taylor, C. E., and Gordon, J. E. (1968): *Interactions of Nutrition and Infection.* WHO Monograph No. 57, Geneva.
31. Tzipori, S., Augus, K. W., Gray, E. W., and Campbell, I. (1981): *Am. J. Vet. Res.*, 42:1400–1404.
32. Vives, M., Mata, L., Castro, B., Simhon, A., and Jimínez, P. (1983): *Rev. Med. Hosp. Nac. Niños (Costa Rica)*, 17:57–70.
33. Wahed, M. A., Rahaman, M. M., Gilman, R. H., Greenough, W. B., and Sarker, S. A. (1981): *ICDDR, B.*, Dacca, Bangladesh. Working Paper No. 22.
34. Whitehead, R. G. (1981): In: *The Impact of Malnutrition on Immune Defense in Parasitic Infestation*, edited by H. Isliker and B. Schurch, pp. 15–25. Hans Huber, Bern.
35. Wyatt, R. G., Yolken, R. H., Urrutia, J. J., Mata, L., Greenberg, H. B., Chanock, R. M., and Kapikian, A. Z. (1979): *Am. J. Trop. Med. Hyg.*, 28:325–328.

Acute Diarrhea: Its Nutritional Consequences in Children, edited by J. A. Bellanti.
Nestlé, Vevey/Raven Press, New York © 1983.

Influence on the Growth Parameters of Children

Discussion

Dr. Klish: I was fascinated to find out, from Dr. Black's data, that *E. coli* was responsible for causing growth failure, in contrast with rotavirus. I would have expected the opposite, since rotavirus seems to produce a disease that causes relatively severe malabsorption of at least the carbohydrates, and *E. coli* tends to produce a disease more attuned to cholera, causing massive malabsorption of fluid and electrolytes but not so much of other nutrients.

Dr. Nalin: I wanted to refer to the fact that in some of the studies from the Center of Vaccine Development with Dr. Levine and others a few years ago, we did show, in volunteers tested before any treatment was given except rehydration fluid, that *E. coli* infections were associated with malabsorption of vitamin A. This persisted after the acute symptoms had subsided. When they were treated several weeks later, the tolerance tests showed that the malabsorption was still there. In areas such as the villages in Bangladesh, I suspect that many of these cases are partially treated or not treated in a way to eradicate the infection, and the possibility of prolonged colonization after the acute attack may be linked with a chronic malabsorption. This may account for long-term effects other than the acute attack.

Dr. Schmidt: In our longitudinal studies we found that the group infected with *E. coli* lost much weight, but that the length of children was very little affected. The reverse was true for children infected with *Shigella.*

Dr. Black: Shigella was fairly consistent in affecting length, both in the short and in the long term. I do not have a ready explanation for the reason why one affects length and the other weight. One might have thought it would be both, and I was somewhat surprised to find an effect with *Shigella*, or that we found it at all.

Dr. Bellanti: Is it not that malnutrition primarily affects weight and not height, unless it is pretty prolonged and severe? This appears to be the opposite.

Dr. Guesry: It seems to me that when we are addressing the question of nutritional consequences of acute diarrhea in children, we should consider both the timing of refeeding of the children and the quality of the food that they are provided. If it is possible to feed the child early after diarrhea because he is still breast-fed, or when you have at your disposal special formulae with easily absorbed fat and adequate protein, the growth may resume rapidly and the period of malnutrition will be short. It is a completely different case when you do not have this possibility.

Dr. Brunser: Every subject who has an episode of diarrhea has a previous history, and in the previous history he may be marked for all the reactions he developed after each episode of diarrhea. In turn, each episode of diarrhea will influence, probably for a long period of time, what will happen later. In Santiago, we are doing a study of people who were apparently healthy. They had no symptoms; they were not excreting any of the known enteropathogens; they were well nourished. There were interesting findings. For example, if you looked at the small intestine, it appeared normal. However, when you put that intestine to work, it did not work properly.

Dr. Bellanti: Were there functional abnormalities?

Dr. Brunser: It had functional abnormalities. For example, lower concentrations of glucose than normal saturated the transport capacity of the intestine of these individuals; the loss of nitrogen through the stools was much greater than in North American, healthy individuals. When you increased the amount of fiber in the food, the loss of nitrogen increased considerably. For a normal child 12 mg/kg/day nitrogen is considered normal. When our subjects received 20 g fiber, the fecal nitrogen went up to 36 or 39 mg/kg/day on an average. The interesting thing was that when we placed these subjects in a metabolic ward and we enforced very strict hygienic conditions for about 3 months, we were able to demonstrate, at least from the morphological point of view, that there was a complete reversal of the morphological changes and the mucosa began to appear like a normal mucosa.

Dr. Bellanti: Were their functional abnormalities reversed also?

Dr. Brunser: Yes. Apparently they are reversed to a considerable extent in about 3 months.

Dr. Mata: When you follow children week by week, you can easily find that about 20% of the *Shigella* infections are chronic. The point is that in dealing with this problem, there are so many variables and *Strongyloides* may be one of them. The only way to make sure that you do not have *Strongyloides* is to do an intubation or a biopsy, and even that may not be enough. There are reported cases of children who went for 6 months without thriving at all, and then repetitive biopsies showed that *Strongyloides* larvae were present and proper treatment cured the parasitism. Thereafter, children started to catch up very quickly.

Dr. Levine: I would like to comment on Dr. Klish's comment that rotavirus does not cause malnutrition and toxigenic *E. coli* does. In a rotavirus infection, the intestinal mucosa is denuded; but the lesion is localized and is in fact surrounded by normal absorbing mucosa. This is the very reason why glucose-electrolyte solution is effective clinically in rotavirus and may in part explain why there is not malnutrition in other absorbing areas. Why does *E. coli* cause malnutrition? We have to remember that although the *E. coli* is toxin-producing, it is not a toxicosis. It is an infection. The *E. coli* must attach themselves and proliferate in the small bowel in order to cause secretory diarrhea. Some years ago we were carrying out studies of gastrointestinal functions with a fairly crude measurement. Individuals were vaccinated with a purified vaccine against a toxigenic *E. coli* organism. The vaccine did not change the intestinal absorption. When they were challenged with toxigenic *E. coli*, there was a striking change in the intestinal absorption in the unvaccinated controls and in those individuals who were protected. The critical thing is that intestinal absorption was significantly changed in the nondiarrheal toxigenic *E. coli* infected people. Even though the toxin was not working because they were protected by the vaccine, just the infection did something to the gut that caused changes. This interaction between the organism and the intestinal mucosa brings in another very important variable that was not mentioned; that is the genetics. Receptors for the organism that allow it to stay in the upper small bowel are very important, and there is evidence from animal and human studies with cholera that the genetic make-up is of consequence in determining the severity of the diarrhea.

Dr. Klish: I would like to respond to Dr. Levine's comment about the patchy lesions of rotavirus. I agree that the rotavirus can cause a patchy lesion, but some of the available data imply that in a large proportion of the cases this lesion is significant enough to cause malabsorption, at least of glucose, in the conventional oral rehydration solution.

Dr. Edelman: Not only is there malabsorption of carbohydrates, but Dr. Muller's group in Bangladesh showed that nitrogen absorption during acute rotavirus diarrhea is substantially depressed compared with *E. coli* and compared with *Shigella*. Fat malabsorption is also more severe in rotavirus than in *E. coli* and *Shigella* infections.

*Acute Diarrhea: Its Nutritional Consequences
in Children*, edited by J. A. Bellanti.
Nestlé, Vevey/Raven Press, New York © 1983.

METABOLIC CONSEQUENCES

Nutritional Metabolic Consequences of Acute Diarrhea in Children

William J. Klish

*Division of Pediatric Gastroenterology and Nutrition, Department of Pediatrics,
University of Rochester Medical Center, Rochester, New York 14627*

Most physicians who treat children with diarrheal illnesses intuitively recognize that diarrhea exerts a profound impact on their nutritional status. These observations are not new. In 1897, L. Emmett Holt (5) wrote in his textbook *Diseases of Infancy and Childhood*: "In infants malnutrition often depends upon some previous acute disease, especially of the stomach and intestines, and sometimes of the lungs."

Interest in quantifying the nutritional impact of infection, in general, began in the 19th century as the science of physiology emerged. It is no surprise that the first observations in host nutritional responses to infection were made in a diarrheal disease. In 1831, O'Shaughnessy (15) measured the stool electrolyte content in patients with acute virulent Asiatic cholera in an effort to understand the pathophysiologic mechanism leading to death in this greatly feared disease. His observations, which were published in The Lancet, quickly led to the first attempts at intravenous replacement of water and electrolytes in cholera by Thomas Latta in 1832 (10). Unfortunately, it took almost a century before this very logical but radical therapy became generally accepted.

During the second half of the 19th century, many of the tools necessary for the study of the metabolic impact of disease on the host emerged. These techniques, which included nitrogen and mineral balance and calorimetry, were immediately applied to a wide variety of infectious illnesses. This work has continued to the present time, and a large body of data has been collected that quantifies the host response to infection. I will attempt to summarize in this chapter the data about the underlying causative mechanisms that permit an infectious process to initiate or produce nutritional deficits in the host. Many of the observations I will make refer to infectious disease as a whole, with the realization that acute diarrhea represents a specific group of infections. As we understand more about the specific etiologies of diarrhea, it is becoming obvious that they exert their influence on the host through a myriad of mechanisms; only some can be reviewed here.

Probably the most dramatic demonstration of the impact of infection on the nutritional status of children was made by Leonardo Mata and his co-

workers (14) and is described in Fig. 1. Shown in this figure is the growth curve
of a single child from birth to 3 years of age who lived in the Guatemalan
village of Santa Maria Cauqué. This child, who was small at birth, followed
an appropriate growth rate until age 6 months, at which time the number of
attacks of infection increased and growth slowed. With the exception of a case
of measles at 9 months of age, every episode of weight loss this child experienced was associated with a bout of diarrhea. Indeed, diarrhea has a profound
impact on the nutritional status of growing children. The weight loss demonstrated in this child resulted from a combination of decreased food intake,
malabsorption of nutrients, and catabolic phenomena that were induced by
the infecting agent.

Fever is a curious physiological phenomenon that occurs in response to
invasion of the body by infectious agents. Most episodes of diarrhea are associated with some degree of fever. It represents an upward displacement of
the core body temperature without disorganization of thermoregulation. Fever
appears to be an evolved pattern of response with survival value. In experiments done by Kluger (9) in poikilothermic lizards, this survival value was
demonstrated. These animals were placed in a chamber with a temperature
gradient. Normal lizards moved to that spot on the chamber floor that allowed

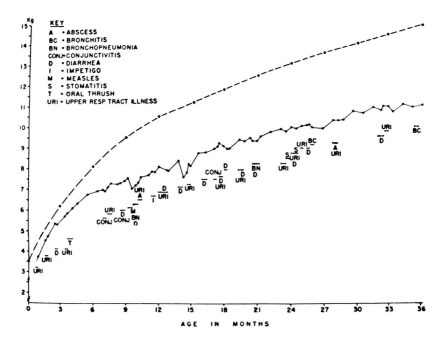

FIG. 1. Illnesses and weight curve of a child from birth to 3 years of age. The *solid line* is the
weight of the child; the *broken line* indicates the median of the Jackson-Kelly standard curve.
The length of the *horizontal lines* indicates the duration of individual episodes of infectious
disease. Note the frequency with which weight loss occurred after bouts of diarrhea and other
infectious diseases.

them to maintain a core temperature of 38.5 to 39°C. When infected with endotoxin from *Aeromonas hydrophila*, these same lizards produced a fever of 2°C by moving to the part of the chamber that resulted in a core temperature of 40 to 41°C. If the lizards were maintained at a constant environmental temperature, the mortality rate varied inversely with the body temperature with 100% mortality at 34°C decreasing to 33% at 40°C.

If this survival value exists in humans, it comes at no small expense. Body temperature results from a balance between heat production and heat loss. DuBois (4) showed in 1937 that to maintain an increase in core temperture of 1°C in adult subjects, a 13% increase in basal metabolic rate was required. This percentage may actually be higher in infants since metabolic rate varies inversely with body size. Malnourished infants may also further increase the metabolic requirements to maintain core temperature, since the loss of subcutaneous fat as an insulating substance would result in more heat loss from the body. In a 9 kg infant whose basal metabolic requirements are 60 kcal/kg/24 hr, one degree of fever would increase caloric requirements by a minimum of about 70 cal/day. As will be discussed later, this increased demand for calories comes at a time when food intake, as well as absorption, is decreased.

Acute infectious illnesses are accompanied by a complex variety of interrelated nutritional and metabolic responses within the host. Very little information about these responses in diarrheal illnesses exists. However, reviewing these events as they occur in other infections can help us understand the full impact of diarrhea. A schematic representation of the sequence of nutritional responses that evolves during the course of a "typical" generalized febrile infectious illness taken from the work of Beisel and his co-workers (1) is shown in Fig. 2. At the moment of exposure, nutrition-related metabolic events begin. The phagocytic activity that takes place requires an increased production of polymorphonuclear cells. This increase in cell turnover quickly reflects itself in a decrease in available substrate, such as amino acids, even before the illness begins. Also, during the incubation period hormonal changes begin to take place. This results in an alteration in the urinary output of certain minerals as though the body were preparing itself for the impending illness. Sodium secretion increases, while phosphate and zinc are retained. At the onset of fever, the secretion of the so-called acute phase serum proteins such as haptoglobin, complement, α_1-antitrypsin, and ceruloplasmin begins. To maintain this synthesis, amino acids are shunted from other protein-requiring mechanisms. As the calorie requirements increase with increasing fever, the body becomes progressively dependent on fat for its metabolic fuel. At the height of the illness, negative balances of many nutrients including nitrogen, potassium, magnesium, and phosphorus begin. The body simultaneously begins to retain salt and water. As the illness subsides, and the hormonal profile returns to normal, diuresis occurs. The return to positive balances of many of the nutrients including nitrogen does not occur for many days into convalescence.

The magnitude of the negative balance for nitrogen is shown in Fig. 3, which is taken from the work of Beisel on sandfly fever and tularemia, and Howard

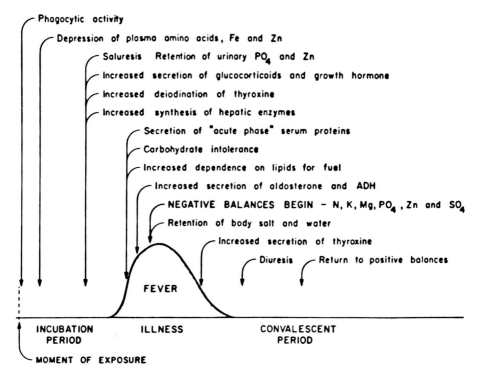

FIG. 2. Schematic representation of the sequence of nutritional responses that evolves during the course of a "typical" generalized febrile infectious illness.

with malaria in 1946 (6). In these studies, adult volunteers were inoculated with the various infective agents and metabolic balance studies carried on throughout the course of the illness. As seen in Fig. 3, the response is the same whether the infective agent is of a virus as in sandfly fever, a bacteria as in tularemia, or a parasite as in malaria. Negative nitrogen balance ensues soon after the fever begins in all three illnesses. In the case of malaria, the amount of nitrogen loss decreases as the disease persists. Obviously, the host is able to adapt to a chronic insult.

A decrease in the intake of nitrogen as well as an increase in the loss of nitrogen in stool and urine could account for a negative balance. To determine what portion of the negative nitrogen balance in tularemia was due to anorexia and a diminished dietary intake, a group of nonexposed control subjects were fed an identical intake as the sick subjects. As shown in Fig. 3, the pair-fed controls developed a negative balance which was only about 30% of that seen in disease, demonstrating that anorexia is only part of the problem. The subjects with tularemia lost an average of about 50 g nitrogen. Since 6.25 g protein equals 1 g nitrogen, these subjects lost 312 g protein. Assuming that all the protein lost was derived from skeletal muscle, and muscle is approximately

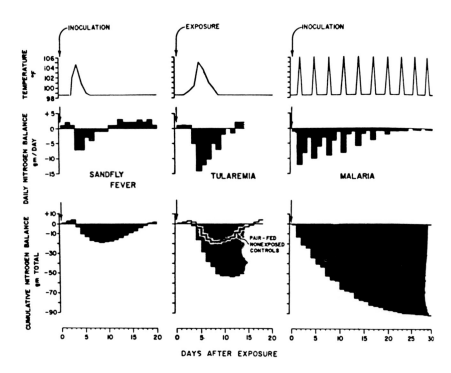

FIG. 3. Nitrogen balance data plotted in relationship to the fever curve in a representative bacterial, viral, and parasitic illness. A cumulative plot of nitrogen balance is also shown for nonexposed controls who were pair-fed to match the tularemia group.

20% protein by weight, these subjects lost an average of 1.5 kg or 3.5 pounds of muscle. This is by no means an insignificant loss and resulted from a disease that lasted only 5 days. It is also of interest to note that it took about 3 weeks before the deficit was recovered. It is no surprise that the Guatemalan child shown earlier who had at least one infectious illness a month failed to thrive.

Negative nitrogen balance can develop even in the absence of fever, as shown in Fig. 4. These data are also taken from the work of Beisel (1) and show a single subject who was exposed to the rickettsial disease, Q fever. The subject developed a subclinical infection and his rectal temperature was never elevated above 100°F, even though rickettsia were present in his blood over an 8-day period. In spite of this, a profound negative nitrogen balance ensued and remained for more than a month.

The nutritional impact of diarrheal illness is compounded by a diminished dietary intake during the disease process. This lack of intake is not only due to anorexia caused by the infection itself, but may be enhanced by the practice of withholding food from children with diarrhea. This practice is particularly prevalent in the developed countries such as the United States, where physicians are frequently taught to continue feeding infants only clear liquids until

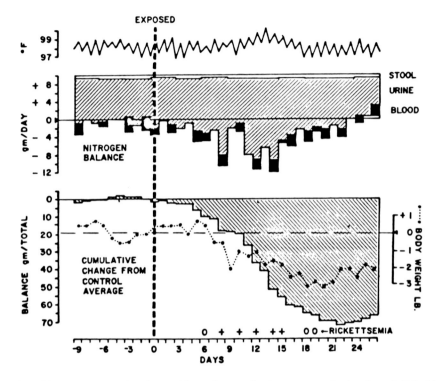

FIG. 4. Nitrogen balance data in a subject who remained asymptomatic despite subclinical Q fever (7). This individual showed neither an elevation of rectal temperature above 100°F nor a diminution of dietary intake despite the presence of *Coxiella burnetii* in the blood over an 8-day period.

the diarrhea has abated. This needless restriction frequently compounds the metabolic impact of diarrheal diseases and results in overt malnutrition.

Data quantifying the impact of diarrheal illness on the dietary intakes of children is very limited. In a longitudinal study by Martorell and co-workers in Guatemala (13), 477 children were observed over a period of about 4 years. Twenty-four-hour dietary recall data were calculated on all children during home visits, and the children were separated into healthy and sick groups based on the presence of selected common symptoms that included diarrhea, vomiting, apathy, fever, and skin rash. Diarrhea and apathy were the two most frequently reported symptoms. The results are shown in Fig. 5 which plots daily caloric intake against age. As shown, the sick children ingested significantly less calories than the healthy children. The reduction in intake was 18% from 15 to 36 months of age, 22% from 42 to 60 months, and 19% across all ages.

In another study done by Hoyle and co-workers (7) in 41 children with acute diarrheal disease hospitalized in a rural treatment center in Bangladesh, the results were similar. After the children were rehydrated, which took an average of 8 hr, the oral intake was measured for one completed 24-hr period. Three groups of children were studied. The first group received routine hospital care, the mothers of the second group received intensive dietary education stressing the importance of feeding, and the third group was made up of healthy control children who accompanied their mothers to the clinic for family planning services. The results are shown in Table 1.

The children with diarrhea ingested 42% less food than the healthy controls. It is interesting to note that training mothers to encourage food intake in their children with diarrhea had no impact on the caloric intake. This suggests that

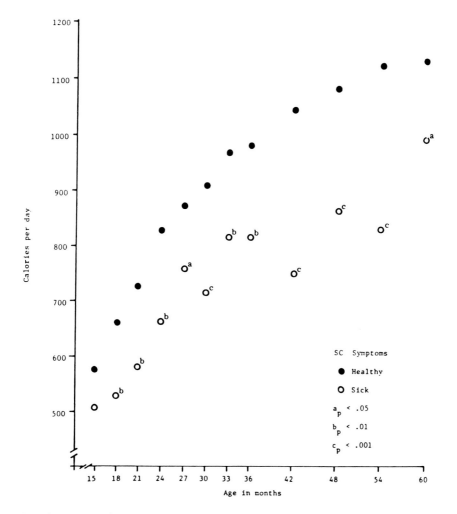

FIG. 5. Comparison of home dietary energy intake for children with or without selected common symptoms (sexes pooled).

TABLE 1. *Total energy intake from breast milk,*
oral fluids, and other foods[a]

		Diarrhea	
Cal/kg/24 hr	Healthy control	No dietary education	Dietary education
Total	129.9 ± 16.8^b	75.0 ± 8.3	60.9 ± 7.4
Breast milk	53.6 ± 6.7	46.9 ± 5.5	49.2 ± 6.2
Oral fluids		10.1 ± 2.0	16.1 ± 2.4
Other foods	86.3 ± 21.1^b	33.3 ± 8.8	12.3 ± 2.6

[a] Total energy intake (cal/kg/24 hr) among control and children with diarrhea.
[b] Statistical significance < 0.05.

anorexia rather than the withholding of food is more important as a cause for the decrease in intake during the early stages of acute diarrhea. It is important to note that the intake of breast milk did not change significantly, implying that breast-feeding is a more effective means of providing adequate intake during diarrhea. Protein intake was similarly affected in this study, dropping from an average of 1.9 g/kg/24 hr to 0.96 g/kg/24 hr.

Even though acute infectious diarrhea interferes with both the intake and utilization of nutrients as described, probably the most profound effect this disease has on the host is that of interfering with the absorption of nutrients. The very term diarrhea implies malabsorption of at least water and electrolytes. Even though the loss of water and electrolytes is most evident clinically, almost all nutrients have been shown to be malabsorbed during acute enteritis. This includes trace elements such as zinc, water-soluble vitamins such as folate and B_{12}, and fat-soluble vitamins such as A, as well as protein, fat, and carbohydrate. It has been estimated that diarrhea may result in an increased calorie loss in stool of as much as 500 to 600 cal/day. Almost every specific diarrheal agent has been shown to be associated with malabsorption including rotavirus and Norwalk virus, bacteria, such as *Salmonella, Shigella,* and *Vibrio cholera,* and protozoans, such as *Giardia lamblia.*

The pathogenesis of malabsorption in patients with diarrheal disease is not well understood for all etiologies. Space also does not permit a review of all the mechanisms postulated. For these reasons, remarks will be confined to the malabsorption of carbohydrates, particularly as it applies to viral gastroenteritis.

Carbohydrate malabsorption is the most problematic absorptive defect caused by acute enteritis, since it not only results in a loss of calories but also prolongs the symptom of diarrhea. When unabsorbed sugars enter the colon, they are fermented by indigenous colonic bacteria to organic acids. These acids can directly interfere with absorptive mechanisms, as well as act as an osmotically active solute that retains water in the lumen of the intestine. Lactose is the most commonly malabsorbed carbohydrate following an episode of acute diarrhea. It is reasonable to expect that the absorption of this sugar would be most easily interfered with, since the enzyme responsible for its hydrolysis and absorption is the least plentiful on the intestinal surface. For every 1 unit of lactase activity present, there are 2 units of sucrase, and 6 to 8 units of maltase.

Two hundred and seventy-one Indian infants with acute diarrhea were studied by Chandrasekaran and co-workers (2) for the presence of carbohydrate intolerance. Only 60 infants had positive bacterial cultures implying that most of the diarrhea was due to virus. Of these infants, 110 or 41% developed carbohydrate malabsorption. Ninety infants had only lactose intolerance, 6 malabsorbed sucrose as well as lactose, and 14 developed total carbohydrate intolerance and protracted diarrhea. Other authors have reported an incidence of carbohydrate intolerance as high as 77%.

It is not difficult to imagine how viral enteritis can result in malabsorption when one examines the effect of the virus on the intestinal mucosa. As shown in Fig. 6, rotavirus causes a significant alteration in the structure of the mucosa. There is marked blunting of the villi associated with an inflammatory reaction in the lamina propria.

The relationship between structure and function of the intestinal tract was investigated by our group several years ago. Infants who developed intractable diarrhea and total carbohydrate intolerance following several episodes of acute gastroenteritis were studied. Intestinal mucosal biopsies were obtained acutely and during convalescence which lasted as long as 5 months. Examples are

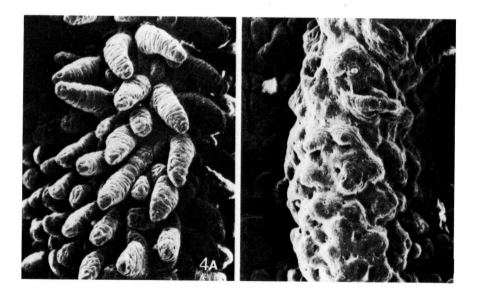

FIG. 6. Scanning electron micrographs of distal small intestine (×45). **A:** Section from control showing slender finger-like villi. **B:** Section from infected piglet at 40 hr. Loss of villi is complete over the folds. Surface openings of crypts appear as pits on the irregular surface.

shown in Fig. 6. Severe villous atrophy was present in the acute stage with partial restoration in the intermediate biopsy. The villi are long in the convalescent biopsy but still not entirely normal, as evidenced by the broad bases and a relative increase in the number of mucous containing cells. During acute disease the microvilli are sparse and severely distorted. The glycocalyx is dispersed into the lumen. During convalescence, the number of microvilli are increased but abnormal tufted forms are prevalent.

These rather dramatic changes in structure undoubtedly alter the functional capacity of the small intestine. To study this relationship as it applies to the absorption of glucose, we devised a method to measure the surface area of a jejunal biopsy using a planographic technique on photographs of multiple sections of biopsies shot under standard magnifications. Just prior to the biopsies, intestinal perfusion studies were done using a nonabsorbable marker to determine the patient's ability to absorb glucose. Both the villous surface as seen under light microscopy, as well as the microvillous surface as seen under electron microscopy, were measured. The total surface area increased during convalescence, as did the rate of glucose absorption from the jejunum. When glucose absorption was plotted against the total surface area as shown in Fig. 7, a significant linear correlation was obtained. These data imply that the alteration in the available surface area becomes a significant limiting factor in the ability of the intestine to absorb carbohydrate.

Certainly there are many more examples of how acute diarrhea can interfere with the nutritional states of the host. To include them all would be impractical. I hope that the examples used have sufficiently highlighted the profound impact a diarrheal illness has upon the host. Not only does it induce a significant malabsorption of nutrients and interfere with the intake of food, but it interferes with the metabolic utilization of these nutrients. Diarrhea

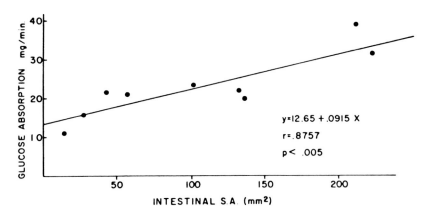

FIG. 7. Total intestinal surface area in mm² over 1 mm² of submucosa plotted against glucose absorption in mg/min/30 cm jejunem. The *points* represent individual studies. The line was determined through linear regression analysis.

undoubtedly represents the single most important health hazard in the world today.

REFERENCES

1. Beisel, W. R. (1977): Magnitude of the host nutritional responses to infection. *Am. J. Clin. Nutr.*, 30:1236.
2. Chandrasekaran, R., Kumar, V., Walia, B. N. S., and Moorthy, B. (1975): Carbohydrate intolerance in infants with acute diarrhea and its complications. *Acta Paediatr. Scand.*, 64:483.
3. Davidson, G. P., and Barnes, G. L. (1979): Structured and functional abnormalities of the small intestine in infants and young children with rotavirus enteritis. *Acta Paediatr. Scand.*, 68:181.
4. DuBois, E. F. (1937): The mechanism of heat loss and temperature regulation. *Lane Medical Lectures.* Stanford University Press, Stanford, California.
5. Holt, L. Emmet (editor) (1897): *The Diseases of Infancy and Childhood.* Appleton, New York.
6. Howard, J. E., Bigham, Jr., and Mason, R. E. (1946): Studies on convalescence. V. Observations on the altered protein metabolism during induced malarial infections. *Trans. Assoc. Am. Physicians*, 59:242.
7. Hoyle, B., Yunus, Md., and Chen, L. C. (1980): Breast feeding and food intake among children with acute diarrheal disease. *Am. J. Clin. Nutr.*, 33:2365.
8. Klish, W. J., Udall, J. N., Rodriguez, J. T., Singer, D. B., and Nichols, B. L. (1978): Intestinal surface area in infant acquired monosaccharide intolerance. *J. Pediatr.*, 92:566.
9. Kluger, M. J., Ringler, D. H., and Anver, M. R. (1975): Fever and survival. *Science*, 188:166.
10. Latta, T. (1832): Letter to the Editor, *Lancet*, 2:274.
11. Lifshitz, F., Coello-Ramnez, P., Gutierrez-Topete, G., and Cornado-Cornet, M. C. (1971): Carbohydrate intolerance in infants with diarrhea. *J. Pediatr.*, 79:760.
12. Lindenbaum, J. (1965): Malabsorption during and after recovery from acute intestinal infection. *Br. Med. J.*, 2:326.
13. Martorell, R., Yarborough, C., Yarborough, S., and Klein, R. E. (1980): The impact of ordinary illnesses on the dietary intakes of malnourished children. *Am. J. Clin. Nutr.*, 33:345.
14. Mata, L., Kromal, R. A., Urrutia, J. J., and Garcia, B. (1977): Effect of infection on food intake and the nutritional state: perspectives as viewed from the village. *Am. J. Clin. Nutr.*, 30:1215.
15. O'Shaugnessy, W. B. (1831): Letter to the Editor. *Lancet*, 1:490.

Acute Diarrhea: Its Nutritional Consequences in Children, edited by J. A. Bellanti.
Nestlé, Vevey/Raven Press, New York © 1983.

METABOLIC CONSEQUENCES

Discussion

Dr. Suskind: If we look at the changes that occur in the host as a result of infection, we see two factors that are playing a role in their nutritional depletion.

One is the effect of the infectious process and the other is the effect of gastroenteritis in terms of malabsorption of nutrients. The combination of the two leads to the clinical and metabolic changes that have been discussed previously.

Infection, whether it is gastroenteritis, pneumonia, or measles, will lead to a reduced intake and anorexia. As a result of the catabolic response to infection, there is an increased loss of nitrogen, potassium, magnesium, zinc, phosphorus, sulphur, vitamins A, C, and B$_2$, and sequestration in the reticuloendothelial system of the following nutrients—iron, copper, and zinc.

Among the endocrine changes, the malnourished child has an increase in growth hormone—an increase in growth hormone that immediately comes down with the first protein meal. In studies that we did in Northern Thailand, growth hormone came down within 2 to 4 hr of the infusion of essential amino acids.

In addition, there is a decrease in insulin and an increase in glucagon in these children. There is also a decrease in T$_3$ and T$_4$, and, in addition, there is an increase in cortisol. If we look at the nutritional consequences of gastroenteritis, we observe a loss of water, sodium, chloride, potassium, and bicarbonate. There is acidemia, but more important, there is a decrease in intestinal absorption.

As a result of infection, therefore, there is a decrease in intake and in absorption of nutrients as well as the catabolic response mentioned earlier. What we have is a clinical state where undernutrition is basically the result of a decreased protein and calorie intake with recurrent episodes of diarrhea leading to a host who is immunologically set up for a more prolonged period of gastroenteritis. This will lead ultimately to marasmic kwashiorkor as a result of the infectious and malabsorption effects of gastroenteritis.

Dr. Black: To go back to the controversy that perhaps I started off by saying which pathogens may be the most important contributors to malnutrition, there may not be as much conflict as it appears. It depends on whether one looks at individual episodes or at a population—I was, in fact, talking about a community of 197 children.

If you look at individual episodes, the evidence right now is equivocal. If we compare individual episodes, the data to which Dr. Edelman referred would indicate that the coefficients of absorption of fat and protein in both rotavirus and *E. coli* are reduced. Likewise, if we look at weight gain, matched episodes of rotavirus and *E. coli* are equivalent. So the data are not yet available to decide on an individual basis which agent is worse. We tried to consider the problem on a population basis. In our study there were 35 episodes of rotavirus and 235 episodes of *E. coli*. *E. coli* had a slightly longer average duration, and we have about a 10-fold difference in the prevalence of days associated with *E. coli* diarrhea compared with rotavirus diarrhea.

Therefore, while we might look at individual episodes and conclude that rotavirus is more severe or has more metabolic consequences, on a population basis, we must consider incidence and prevalence and duration. If we look at individual episodes of rotavirus, *E. coli*, or shigellosis, rotavirus is the one that is most commonly associated with fever. But on a population basis, if you look at all days of fever, more of them are associated with shigellosis and/or with *E. coli* than with rotavirus. Therefore, I don't think there is necessarily a conflict.

Dr. Suskind: I have one question for the gastroenterologists and infectious disease specialists. What is the effect of undernutrition on gastric secretion and on mucus production in the intestine; how does it affect the ability of the host to handle microorganisms that would ordinarily not be populating the small bowel?

Dr. Klish: Concerning the effect of malnutrition on some of the physiological aspects of bowel function, there is unequivocal evidence that there is a decrease in gastric secretion during malnutrition and relative achlorhydria; this obviously would allow a larger number of infective bacteria to get through the stomach and affect the bowels. If 2 infants, a malnourished and a normal one, were subjected to the same infecting dose, the malnourished one should have a greater effect from it. There is also a question regarding the motility of the bowel. If the bowel is malnourished, it may have decreased muscular function, resulting in impaired peristaltism.

This probably happens because a large proportion of malnourished children have contaminated upper small bowels, implying that the cleansing effect of peristaltism, which is important in keeping the upper small bowel sterile, is impaired. Malnourished infants therefore are more susceptible to infectious agents.

Dr. Sabra: We have been working with malnourished children and I think the loss of mucus is a very important thing that plays a role in the bacterial overgrowth. Malnourished children have more bacteria than do normal children.

Acute Diarrhea: Its Nutritional Consequences in Children, edited by J. A. Bellanti.
Nestlé, Vevey/Raven Press, New York © 1983.

BOVINE MILK IMMUNOGLOBULINS

Potential Use of Bovine Milk Immunoglobulins

*C. Mietens, †H. Hilpert, and *H. Werchau

Westfälische Landeskinderklinik-Universitätsklinik und Institut für Medizinische Mikrobiologie und Virologie der Ruhr-Universität, Bochum, Federal Republic of Germany; and †Research Department, Nestlé Products Technical Assistance Company, Ltd., Vevey, Switzerland

In the etiology of acute diarrhea in infancy, bacterial and viral agents play an equally important role (L. Mata, *this volume*). It seems essential to develop adequate measures for the prevention and treatment of these infections. One possible treatment of acute bacterial enteritis, especially those infections caused by enteropathogenic *Escherichia coli*, is by oral administration of bovine milk immunoglobulins with specific antibody activity against these infectious agents. Such bovine milk immunoglobulin concentrates (MIC) have already been prepared and successfully tested in human infants (1,4,6).

ANTI-*E. COLI* MIC: BRIEF DESCRIPTION OF PREPARATION

Pregnant cows were immunized during the last 6 to 8 weeks of gestation by repeated s.c. and i.v. injections of a polyvalent *E. coli* vaccine (see Table 1 for composition). Appropriate volumes of diluted vaccine were infused into the mammary gland through the 4 teat channels 4 and 5 weeks before calving. MIC was isolated from the first 16 milkings of these immunized cows as previously described (4). The average chemical composition of MIC is presented in Table 2, while its immunobiological activity as measured by passive hemagglutination, bacteriostatic activity, phagocytic *in vivo* clearance, and a mouse protection test is presented in Table 3.

CLINICAL STUDIES WITH ANTI-*E. COLI* MIC

Sixty infants hospitalized at the Westfälische Landeskinderklinik–Universitätsklinik-Bochum with acute gastroenteritis and positive stool cultures for enteropathogenic *E. coli* were included in this study. In addition to the usual dietary regimen and the administration of parenteral fluids, if necessary, these children received 1 g MIC/kg body wt/day *per os* equally distributed over all meals. The usual duration of this treatment was 10 days. Stool cultures

TABLE 1. *Serotypes of enteropathogenic* E. coli *included in the vaccine used for immunization of pregnant cows*

O18:K76 (B20)	O112:K66 (B11)
O20:K17 (1)	O119:K69 (B14)
O26:K60 (B6)	O124:K72 (B17)
O44:K74 (L)	O125:K70 (B15)
O55:K59 (B5)	O126:K71 (B16)
O86:K61 (B7)	O127:K63 (B8)
O111:K58 (B4)	O128:K67 (B12)

TABLE 2. *Analysis of milk immunoglobulin concentrate (MIC)*

Composition	%	%
Total protein content		80 ± 5
Immunoglobulins	40 ± 5	
IgG_1 (approximately 75%)		
IgG_2 (approximately 3%)		
IgA (approximately 17%)		
IgM (approximately 6%)		
α-Lactalbumin	15 ± 5	
β-Lactoglobulin	35 ± 5	
Serum albumin	3 ± 2	
Other proteins	7 ± 2	
Humidity		4 ± 0.5
Lactose		3 ± 1
Mineral salts		5 ± 2
Nonprotein nitrogen		7 ± 2

TABLE 3. *Immunobiological activity of anti-*E. coli *MIC*

Bacterial passive hemagglutination
  Titers of a 0.5% MIC solution varied between 1:64 and 1:256 against the different *E. coli* serotypes

Bacteriostatic activity (*in vitro*)
  10 μg anti-*E. coli* MIC/ml inhibited growth of 1.5×10^3 bacteria/ml for up to 4 hr

Phagocytic clearance (*in vivo*)
  2.5×10^6 *E. coli* O111:B4 + 10 μg anti-*E. coli* MIC injected i.v. into mice resulted in 99.6% clearance of bacteria from blood within 20 min.

Protection test in mice[a]
  Protection with 20 μg anti-*E. coli* MIC against 10×1 LD_{100} *E. coli* O111:B4

[a] Control: no protection with 100 μg MIC from nonimmunized cows.

were performed on days 3, 6, 9, 12, 13, and 14 after starting MIC treatment. The treatment was considered effective only if all three cultures, after termination of MIC administration (days 12, 13, and 14), were negative. Some children had to be treated with antibiotics for intercurrent infections.

Fifty-one patients had stool cultures yielding *E. coli* serotypes which were included in the vaccine used for the preparation of MIC. The results are summarized in Table 4.

A smaller group of 9 children had stool cultures positive for *E. coli* serotypes which had not been included in the vaccine (see Table 5). These infants served as a control group. From 51 patients in the first group, 43 (84.3%) had negative stool cultures after treatment with MIC, although 4 required two treatment cycles to eliminate the enteropathogenic *E. coli*. In 8 patients (15.7%), the stool cultures remained positive.

In the control group, only 1 patient became negative while the stools of 8 infants remained positive with *E. coli*. The differences between the test group and the control group are highly significant (see Table 6). These results remain unchanged whether patients receiving antibiotic treatment for intercurrent respiratory infections (ampicillin or cephalotin) were included in the analyses or not. From these studies we can conclude that orally administered specific anti-*E. coli* bovine milk immunoglobulins are statistically effective in the treatment of infantile *E. coli* gastroenteritis.

POTENTIAL USE OF MIC FOR TREATMENT OF ROTAVIRUS INFECTIONS

In recent years it has been shown that 40 to 60% of all cases of gastroenteritis during infancy are caused by rotavirus infections (3,5,8). For this reason we

TABLE 4. *Results of treatment with bovine milk-Ig concentrate containing antibodies to isolated* E. coli *serotypes[a]*

E. coli serotype	No. of infants	Results of treatment[b]	
		Effective	Noneffective
O111:K58 (B4)	18	14 (5)	4
O55:K59 (B5)	4	4 (1)	—
O26:K60 (B6)	4	4	—
O128:K67 (B12)	6	6	—
O86:K61 (B7)	1	1 (1)	—
O127:K63 (B8)	3	3	—
O125:K70 (B15)	7	4 (3)	3 (1)
O126:K71 (B16)	2	2	—
O119:K69 (B14)	1	—	1 (1)
O44:K74 (L)	5	5 (1)	—
Total	51	43 (11)	8 (2)

[a] *n* = 51.
[b] Numbers of patients receiving antibiotics appear in brackets.

TABLE 5. *Results of treatment with bovine milk-Ig concentrate containing no antibodies to isolated* E. coli *serotypes[a]*

E. coli serotypes	No. of infants	Results of treatment[b]	
		Effective	Noneffective
O78:K80 (B—)	8	1 (1)	7 (3)
O114:K— (B—)	1	—	1
Total	9	1 (1)	8 (3)

[a] $n = 9$.
[b] Numbers of patients receiving antibiotics appear in brackets.

investigated the frequency of rotavirus infections among the children admitted with diarrhea to our hospital (see Fig. 1). The figures represent the monthly numbers of rotavirus infections during the last 2 years. The seasonal prevalence of rotavirus infection is evident with a peak from November to April.

Figure 2 reviews the age of the affected infants. The majority of patients were young infants mainly between 4 and 8 months. After the age of 12 months there was a sharp decrease in the attack rate. Table 7 shows the incidence of clinical symptoms. Diarrhea, vomiting, and fever were observed most frequently; 66% had respiratory symptoms and 39% had severe dehydration.

Diarrhea (Fig. 3) lasted for 2 to 8 days with a mean of 4 to 6 days. Fever (Fig. 4) lasted 2 to 4 days; in a few patients it lasted somewhat longer. The most frequently observed temperatures were between 38° and 39°C.

Vomiting (Fig. 5) occurred most frequently during the first 2 to 4 days. The persistence of viruses in the stools varied considerably (Fig. 6). Most patients

TABLE 6. *Statistical analysis of MIC treatment[a]*

Group	Treatment		Total
	Effective	Noneffective	
All patients ($n = 60$)[a]			
Group 1	43 (84.3%)	8 (15.7%)	51
Group 2	1	8	9
Total	44	16	60
Patients not receiving antibiotics ($n = 43$)[b]			
Group 1	32 (84.2%)	6 (15.8%)	38
Group 2	0	5	5
Total	32	11	43

[a] $\chi^2 = 15.8193$; df $= 1$; $p < 0.01$.
[b] $\chi^2 = 12.3228$; df $= 1$; $p < 0.01$.

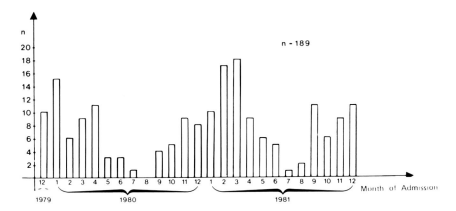

FIG. 1. Seasonal distribution of admission of children with rotavirus infections over a 2-year period.

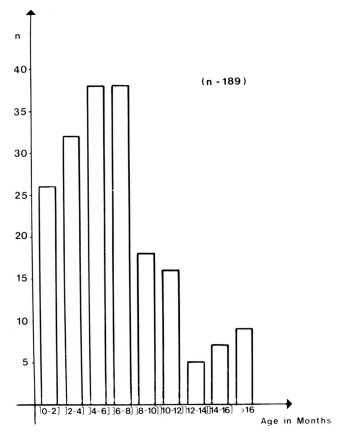

FIG. 2. Age distribution of children with rotavirus infections.

TABLE 7. *Symptomatology of infants*
with rotavirus infection[a]

Symptom	No.	%
Diarrhea	178	98.9
Vomiting	158	87.8
Fever	146	81.1
Respiratory tract disease	115	65.8
Dehydration	68	38.8

[a] $n = 180$.

excreted viruses for 6 to 8 days, but some did excrete viruses up to the 12th day after the initial symptoms.

The question arose as to if there was a relation between the length of virus excretion and the clinical symptoms. Chi square-test analysis revealed a good correlation between the duration of virus excretion and (a) fever, (b) diarrhea, and (c) vomiting. This indicates that patients should be considered infectious at least as long as these signs persist. On the other hand, virus excretion is also closely related to the severity of the disease. The impact of rotavirus infection

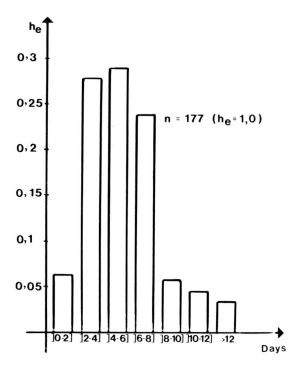

FIG. 3. Relative frequency (h_e) of duration of diarrhea in rotavirus infection.

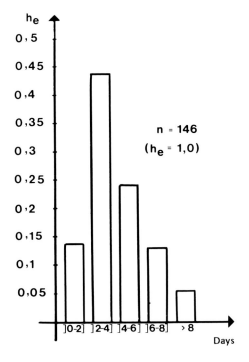

FIG. 4. Relative frequency (h_e) of duration of elevated temperatures in rotavirus infection.

on water and electrolyte balance was considerable in most patients; 17 patients showed hyperosmolarity, while 6 showed hypoosmolarity (Fig. 7). The concentration of blood electrolytes is shown in Fig. 8. Quite a number of patients had hyponatremia and hypochloremia, and those with hyperosmolarity usually showed elevated blood urea values. All patients recovered with carefully controlled fluid and electrolyte substitution.

We can conclude that rotavirus infections are a major etiologic factor of infantile diarrhea in moderate climate zones during the cold season. Considerable dehydration and electrolyte imbalance may develop.

Our efforts must be directed to find effective methods for treatment and prevention of this disease. Theoretically four approaches could be envisaged.

1. Administration of virostatics: A considerable number of substances inhibiting viral replication *in vitro* are known and some of them might inhibit rotavirus as well. However, clinical application is limited by cellular toxicity. The critical point is to reach a high enough concentration in the cells to block the production of ribonucleic acid (RNA) and viral proteins without interfering with normal cell metabolism. At present no effective anti-rotavirus drug is available and it seems questionable if there will be one in the near future.

2. Active vaccination: As passively transferred maternal serum antibodies seem to have only little protective effect against rotavirus infection in young

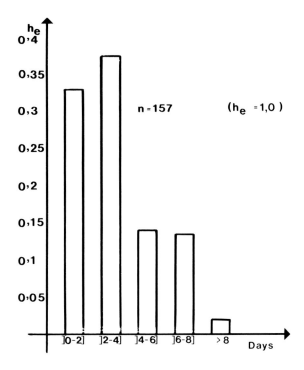

FIG. 5. Relative frequency (h_e) of duration of vomiting in rotavirus infection.

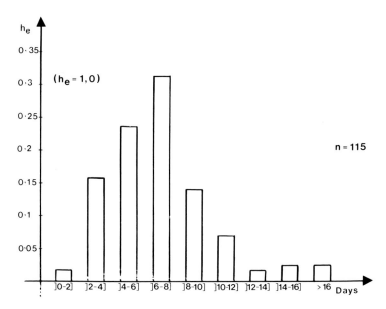

FIG. 6. Relative frequency (h_e) of duration of virus excretion following initial symptoms in rotavirus infection.

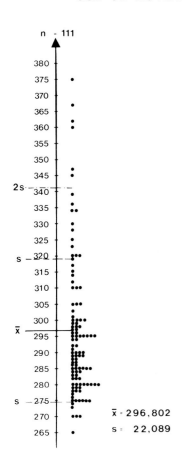

FIG. 7. Distribution of blood osmolarity (in mOsm/kg) in patients with rotavirus infection.

$\bar{x}$ = 296,802

s = 22,089

infants, the formation of local immunity on the intestinal mucosa seems essential for its prevention. This can only be achieved by active immunization with a live attenuated human rotavirus strain. Propagation of rotavirus on cell culture was successful (T. Konno, *this volume*; ref. 7), but propagation of larger amounts of human rotavirus is still problematic. Furthermore, it will probably take some time to clone a well-attenuated and stable strain suitable for vaccine production on a larger scale. Although there are still many difficulties to overcome, the best protection against rotavirus infection will most probably be through active immunization, at least for the older infants (>6 months). Meanwhile, we must find another treatment for these infants and for those who cannot be immunized.

3. Administration of specific human immunoglobulins: As outlined above, antibodies to rotavirus will be effective only when secreted locally or after oral application. For successful treatment or prophylaxis, large amounts of human hyperimmune gammaglobulins would be needed. Some results of treatment with serum gammaglobulins have been presented (2). With regard to the nec-

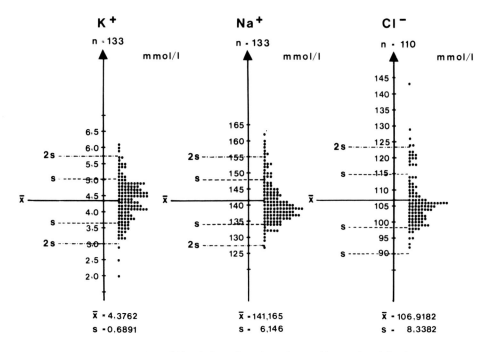

FIG. 8. Distribution of blood electrolytes in patients with rotavirus infection.

essary quantities of blood serum gammaglobulins and its elevated price this way of treatment or prevention seems rather impractical.

4. Administration of specific bovine milk immunoglobulins: A promising and feasible way in the near future could be the application of bovine milk immunoglobulins with high anti-rotavirus antibody activity. They could be used for treatment and prophylaxis. Rotavirus infections are of an epizootic character in cows and most of them secrete milk with a high anti-rotavirus antibody titer in their colostral phase. As bovine and human rotavirus strains share common antigens, a MIC with high anti-bovine rotavirus antibody activity has been prepared from this milk.

Based on the promising results obtained with the anti-*E. coli* MIC, we are now carrying out clinical trials with this material to determine its effectiveness in the prophylaxis and treatment of human rotavirus infections.

REFERENCES

1. Ballabriga, A., Farriaux, J. P., Hilpert, H., Gerber, H., and Arcalis, L. (1976): Specific anti-*E. coli* bovine milk immunoglobulins in the treatment of infants with intestinal *E. coli* infections. *Acta Paediatr. Belg.*, 29:126.
2. Barnes, G. L., Hewson, P. H., and McLellan, J. A. (1982): Randomized trial of oral gammaglobulin in low-birth-weight infants infected with rotavirus. *Lancet*, 1/8286:1371.

3. Blacklow, N. R., and Cukor, G. (1981): Viral gastroenteritis. *N. Engl. J. Med.,* 304:397.
4. Hilpert, H., Gerber, H., Amster, H., Pahud, J. J., Ballabriga, A., Arcalis, L., Farriaux, J. P., de Peyer, E., and Nusslé, D. (1977): Bovine milk immunoglobulins (Ig), their possible utilisation in industrially prepared infant milk formulae. In: *Food and Immunology. Swedish Nutrition Foundation Symposium XIII,* edited by L. Hambraeus, L. A. Hanson, and H. McFarlane, p. 182. Almquist and Wiksell, Stockholm.
5. Kapikian, A. Z., Kim, H. W., Wyatt, R. G., Cline, W. L., Arrobio, J. D., Brandt, C. D., Rodriquez, W. J., Sack, D. A., Canock, R. M., and Parrott, R. H. (1976): Human reovirus-like agent as the major pathogen associated with "winter" gastroenteritis in hospitalized infants and young children. *N. Engl. J. Med.,* 294:965.
6. Mietens, C., Kleinhorst, H., Hilpert, H., Gerber, H., Amster, H., and Pahud, J. J. (1979): Treatment of infantile *E. coli* gastroenteritis with specific bovine anti-*E. coli* milk immunoglobulins. *Eur. J. Pediatr.,* 132:239.
7. Sato, K., Inaba, Y., Shinozaki, T., Fujii, R., and Matumoto, M. (1981): Isolation of human rotavirus in cell cultures. *Arch. Virol.,* 69:155.
8. Steinhoff, M. C. (1980): Rotavirus: The first five years. *J. Pediatr.,* 96:611.

Acute Diarrhea: Its Nutritional Consequences in Children, edited by J. A. Bellanti.
Nestlé, Vevey/Raven Press, New York © 1983.

BOVINE MILK IMMUNOGLOBULINS

Comments

H. Hilpert and H. Link-Amster

Research Department, Nestlé Products Technical Assistance Company, Ltd., Vevey, Switzerland

IMMUNOBIOLOGICAL ADAPTATION OF INFANT MILK FORMULAE

The superiority of human milk for the nutrition of the newborn and young infant is not only based on its well-balanced composition by which the infant's nutritional requirements are met, but also on the presence of various immune and nonimmune factors (Table 1) that contribute to build up—*ex alimentatione*—infant resistance against infectious diseases and/or allergic disorders.

Over a long period, infant milk formulae were prepared to achieve the same composition as that of human milk. This led to formulae that were satisfactory to the young infant from a nutritional point of view. However, until now, no specific or nonspecific resistance-enhancing factors could be incorporated into such formulae. We therefore examined the possibilities of their "immunobiological adaptation."

As there is much evidence that human milk immunoglobulins (Ig) with specific antibody activity play an important role in local host defense in the infant's digestive tract, we tested to find if the role of human milk Ig could be played by bovine milk Ig by introducing them into cow's milk formulae.

HUMAN MILK IG VERSUS BOVINE MILK IG

The immunobiological role of human and bovine milk Ig differs considerably. The human infant is born with a prenatally acquired humoral immunity and the Ig present in human milk are predominantly composed of secretory IgA which are practically not absorbed. IgA show a remarkable resistance against digestion by proteolytic enzymes and are thus able to exert an antibody activity in the gut lumen and its mucosal surface.

The calf is born with no significant humoral immunity, characterized by a virtually complete absence of Ig in the newborn blood serum. The offspring receives maternal antibody by oral ingestion of colostral milk which is rich in Ig. Absorption of maternal Ig occurs across the intestinal mucosa during the

TABLE 1. *Protective factors in human milk*

For specific protection
    Immunoglobulins with specific antibody activity (Iga, IgG, IgM)
    Living leukocytes (mainly macrophages, some lymphocytes)
For general unspecific protection
    Lysozyme
    Lactoferrin
    Factor anti-staphylococci (in milk fat)
    Complement factors C_3 and C_4
    Glycoproteins with *N*-acetylneuraminic acid
    Growth factor for *Lactobacillus bifidus*
    Lactoperoxidase

first 36 hr after birth (see Fig. 1). Qualitatively, bovine and human milk contain the same Ig classes (IgG, IgM, and IgA), but there are large quantitative differences (see Fig. 2). In human milk, secretory IgA is the predominant Ig class, whereas IgG_1 is by far the most abundant Ig in bovine mammary secretions.

These differences between human and bovine milk Ig had to be examined carefully before deciding to use bovine milk Ig in infant nutrition.

FIVE CRITERIA FOR THE POTENTIAL USE OF BOVINE MILK IG

Petersen and Campbell (8) were the first to propose the use of cow's milk antibodies for passive oral immunization. But while these authors claimed to induce a general humoral immunity by resorption of milk antibodies through the intestinal wall, our concept is based on the assumption that bovine milk Ig play a similar role to that of human secretory IgA by imparting local passive immunity to the infant's gut.

Five criteria have to be satisfied to comply with this requirement. These are as follows:

1. Bovine milk Ig must display at least part of the antibody specificity which is normally found in human milk Ig.

The induction of specific antibody activity in bovine milk Ig is relatively simple. To obtain high antibody concentrations in cow's milk, pregnant cows were hyperimmunized in the final phase of gestation and during their late lactation period. Potential antigens for immunization are infectious agents in infantile gastroenteritis such as enteropathogenic and enterotoxigenic *E. coli*, cholera enterotoxin, campylobacters, rotaviruses, and other enteroviruses. To overcome the problems linked with serotype specificity of microorganisms, we also envisage immunizing with virulence factors such as enterotoxins and colonization factors. It is clear that the very large spectrum of tailor-made specific antibodies found in human milk is hardly attainable.

2. The antibody activity must be preserved during processing.

The antibody-containing milk cannot be submitted to normal heat treatment to assure bacteriological safety. Absence of viral and bacterial contam-

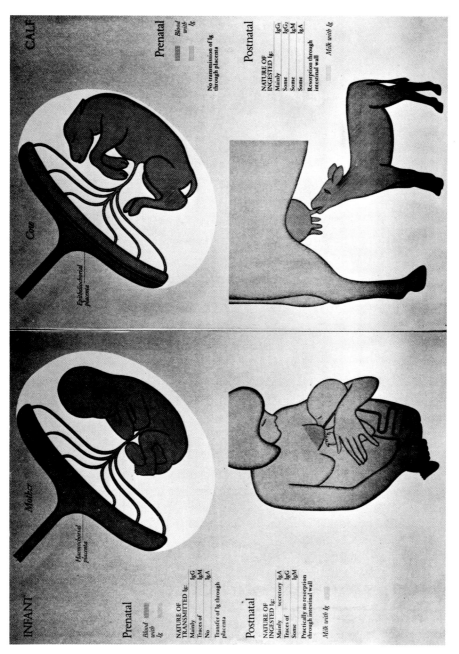

FIG. 1. Schematic comparison of pre- and postnatal transmission of passive immunity in man and cow.

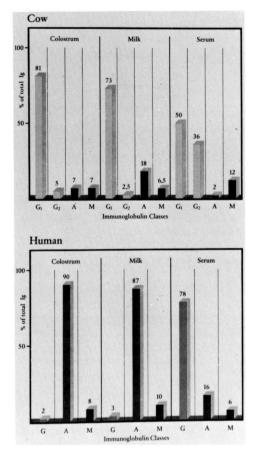

FIG. 2. Relative percentage of Ig in mammary secretions and in blood serum of humans and cows. (From ref. 2.)

ination was achieved by a low temperature treatment (+56°C, 30 min) and sterile filtration of the casein-free lactoserum. The bulk of lactose and mineral salts was removed in a reverse osmosis system. The resulting milk Ig concentrate (MIC) contains 30 to 40% milk Ig after drying at temperatures not higher than +60°C, and exhibits the same antibody activity as the original milk.

3. The specific bovine milk antibodies must show protective activity by interfering with the pathomechanism of enteropathogenic microorganisms.

Immunobiological activity of anti-*E. coli* MIC was demonstrated *in vitro* by passive hemagglutination, bacterial agglutination, and bacterial growth inhibition. *In vivo* antimicrobial activity was proven by phagocytic clearance of opsonized *E. coli* and protection tests in mice (5,9). Inactivation of *E. coli* enterotoxin was shown in the rabbit ileal loop method (10) and by the inhibition of morphological changes in Y-1 cell cultures (H. Link-Amster, *unpublished*). Bacterial adherence to isolated cells from rabbit intestinal mucosa was inhibited by MIC (3). Finally, incubation of enteropathogenic *E. coli* with anti-*E. coli* MIC resulted in the elimination of virulence in mice, probably by a selection of mutants with repressed virulence (7). Anti-rotavirus MIC was tested *in vitro* by enzyme-linked immunosorbent assay (ELISA) and a virus neutralization test.

4. The bovine milk antibodies should resist inactivation by proteolytic degradation during gastrointestinal passage.

Similar to human secretory IgA, bovine milk-Ig (73–81% IgG_1) withstand proteolytic digestion to a considerable extent (4). Extracts from stools of infants who had been given anti-*E. coli* MIC showed intact Ig and active IgG_1-fragment $F(ab')_2$ (5). It is assumed that antibodies which display activity in stool extracts must have been active while passing through the intestine.

5. The prophylactic and therapeutic value of a milk formula enriched with specific milk antibodies must be established by comprehensive laboratory and clinical trials.

The clinical efficiency of anti-*E. coli* MIC in treatment and prevention of infantile *E. coli* gastroenteritis has been shown (1,6), but the question remains open whether rotavirus gastroenteritis in infants can be prevented or treated with anti-rotavirus MIC. Although there is some immunological relationship between bovine and human rotaviruses, *in vitro* neutralization of human rotavirus with anti-bovine rotavirus milk antibodies occurs only at high antibody concentrations. Antibodies directed against the human rotaviruses should have a higher neutralizing activity. Since some human rotaviruses can now be propagated in cell culture, the preparation of corresponding MIC is in progress. It will soon be submitted to clinical testing.

CONCLUDING REMARKS

Breast-feeding is the optimal nutrition for the newborn and the young infant. The nutritional and immunological properties of human milk will probably never be equaled even by the most sophisticated formulae.

Bovine milk-Ig with specific antibody activity can only have restricted application in infant formulae primarily because of their limited availability. The bovine mammary gland seems to be a source of abundant quantities of milk antibodies, but the necessity to specifically hyperimmunize milking cows and to apply a particular technological treatment are the reasons for these limitations. Moreover, for the majority of bottle-fed infants growing up under normal hygienic conditions, infection with enteropathogens is not a serious health threat. The infant population which would gain the greatest benefit from MIC-supplemented formulae is the infant at risk. This comprises the preterm infant, low-birth-weight infants, hospitalized infants, and infants living under precarious hygienic conditions.

REFERENCES

1. Ballabriga, A., Farriaux, J. P., Hilpert, H., Gerber, H., Arcalis, L. (1976): Specific anti-*E. coli* bovine milk immunoglobulins in the treatment of infants with intestinal *E. coli* infections. *Acta Paediatr. Belg.*, 29:126.

2. Butler, J. E. (1974): In: *Lactation*, Vol. 3, edited by B. L. Larson and V. R. Smith, p. 217. Academic Press, New York.
3. Demierre, G., Rivier, D., Hilpert, H., Gerber, H., and Zinkernagel, R. (1975): Adherence of pathogenic *E. coli* to epithelial cells isolated from the intestinal mucosa of the rabbit. *Pathol. Microbiol.*, 42:137–146.
4. de Rham, O., and Isliker, H. (1977): Proteolysis of bovine immunoglobulins. *Int. Arch. Allergy Appl. Immunol.*, 55:61–69.
5. Hilpert, H., Gerber, H., Amster, H., Pahud, J. J., Ballabriga, A., Arcalis, L., Farriaux, J. P., de Peyer, E., and Nusslé, D. (1977): Bovine milk immunoglobulins (Ig), their possible utilization in industrially prepared infant's milk formulae. In: *Food and Immunology, Swedish Nutrition Foundation Symposium XIII*, edited by L. Hambraeus, L. A. Hanson, and H. McFarlane, pp. 182–196. Almquist and Wiksell, Stockholm.
6. Mietens, C., Kleinhorst, H., Hilpert, H., Gerber, H., Amster, H., and Pahud, J. J. (1979): Treatment of infantile *E. coli* gastroenteritis with specific bovine anti-*E. coli* milk immunoglobulins. *Eur. J. Pediatr.*, 132:239–252.
7. Pahud, J. J., Hilpert, H., Schwarz, K., Amster, H., and Smiley, M. (1981): Bovine milk antibodies in the treatment of enteric infections and their ability to eliminate virulence factors from pathogenic *E. coli*. In: *The Ruminant Immune System*, edited by J. E. Butler, pp. 591–600. Plenum, New York.
8. Petersen, W. E., and Campbell, B. (1955): Use of protective principles in milk and colostrum in prevention of disease in men and animals. *J.-Lancet, Minneapolis*, 75:494–496.
9. Rivier, D., and Sobotka, J. (1978): Protective effect of rabbit immune serum administered orally to rats infected by a human pathogenic strain of *E. coli*. *Exp. Cell Biol.*, 46:277–288.
10. Zinkernagel, R., and Colombini, A. (1975): Passive oral immunization with bovine immunoglobulins: Enteropathogenic *E. coli* from infants and bovine anti-*E. coli* lactoserum assayed in the rabbit ileal loop model. *Med. Microbiol. Immunol.*, 162:1–7.

Acute Diarrhea: Its Nutritional Consequences in Children, edited by J. A. Bellanti. Nestlé, Vevey/Raven Press, New York © 1983.

Bovine Milk Immunoglobulins

Discussion

Dr. Bellanti: I would like to ask Dr. Hilpert whether in the preparation of his material, the bacterial extracts were injected intramuscularly or were they given locally into the cow's udder?

Dr. Hilpert: It was a combined immunization, locally into the udder and intramuscularly.

Dr. Bellanti: Do you find a greater concentration of antibody in the cow's milk when it's given locally versus systemically?

Dr. Hilpert: There is no difference as far as the colostrum is concerned. But in the following period, it is necessary to have a local immunization.

Dr. Chandra: I would like to ask Dr. Hilpert about two possible consequences of using a preparation to which sensitization or immune response might develop. First, if you used the same preparation on a number of occasions and in the same child, did you look for a more rapid clearance? Because some of it, I expect, would be absorbed and would induce sensitization, which subsequently would induce faster clearance. Second, was any adverse effect related to, for instance, the bovine globulin part of the preparation?

Dr. Hilpert: We did not observe any kind of negative reaction in these infants as far as they could be followed.

Dr. Bellanti: The point that is being raised here, however, is a very important one, i.e., the whole issue of the role of macromolecular penetration of proteins in a bowel that has been damaged essentially by diarrhea. There is evidence now that there is a greater absorption of macromolecules and proteins in such children who are milk-fed; this may lead to allergic consequences.

*Acute Diarrhea: Its Nutritional Consequences
in Children*, edited by J. A. Bellanti.
Nestlé, Vevey/Raven Press, New York © 1983.

Malnutrition and Immunocompetence: An Overview

R. K. Chandra

*Department of Pediatric Research, Memorial University of Newfoundland, and
Department of Immunology, Janeway Child Health Centre, St. John's,
Newfoundland, Canada*

> To a man with an empty stomach,
> food is God.
>
> *Mahatma Gandhi (1862–1948)*

The association between famine and pestilence has been recorded in ancient history. Puranic literature and biblical references cite observations that suggest an increase in the prevalence and severity of infection among starved individuals and populations. Besides these historic observations, several types of evidence may be marshalled to support causal links between malnutrition, impaired immunity, and infectious illness.

EVIDENCE FOR CAUSAL INTERACTION BETWEEN MALNUTRITION, IMPAIRED IMMUNITY, AND INFECTION

Epidemiologic studies document increased mortality and morbidity in infants and young children with protein-energy malnutrition (PEM). In rural India, the probability of death among young children increases progressively with deterioration in nutritional status (Table 1). Most of the deaths are due to infectious illness and diarrheal illness. The attack rate as well as duration of diarrhea are increased in the malnourished (Table 2). The severity of infectious diseases is also increased in PEM. The most cited examples are measles and herpes simplex virus. There is, however, an unexplained difference in the natural history of measles in PEM in West Africa and Eastern India. There also is an impression among clinicians working in developing countries that common pyogenic infections are more common and severe in malnourished children. The prevalence of PEM among children with lymphoreticular malignancy complicated with *Pneumocystis carinii* infection is higher than in those without such infection (Table 3). Similar data are available for adults undergoing surgery in North American hospitals (Table 4). Finally, the pattern of organisms isolated from malnourished children resembles the findings in

TABLE 1. *Risk of death by nutritional status in infants in rural India[a]*

Weight-for-height (% standard)	Mortality rate (%)
> 80	0.45
71–80	2.16
61–70	9.87
< 60	18.14

[a] Infants were aged 1 to 23 months.

patients with primary defects of immunity (Table 5), thereby pointing to the possible link between PEM, impaired immunocompetence, and infection.

Confounding Variables

Many studies conducted in the last 15 years have addressed the question of immunocompetence in PEM. Host defence is a composite protective umbrella consisting of antigen-specific mechanisms (Fig. 1) (immunoglobulin-antibody system, cell-mediated immunity) and nonspecific mechanisms (skin, mucous membranes, cilia, mucus, interferon, macrophages and microphages, complement system, etc.). Defect in one facet, e.g., phagocytes, as seen in inherited chronic granulomatous disease, may produce serious life-threatening disease, whereas in another instance, e.g., selective IgA deficiency, it may be asymptomatic. PEM produces many rents in the protective umbrella; even though a single defect may not be sufficient to increase susceptibility to disease, each deficit probably has an additive, even synergistic, effect.

At the same time, it must be pointed out that there are many confounding variables that impinge on the nutrition-immunity-infection nexis. Some of these are highlighted here.

1. Coexistent but unrecognized deficiencies of other nutrients are frequently present in PEM. Each of these nutrients may exert an important influence on immune response.

TABLE 2. *Diarrhea morbidity*

Weight-for-height (% standard)	Episodes of diarrhea per 12 months	Duration of episode (days)
> 80	3.0 ± 0.4[a]	3.1 ± 0.8
< 80	6.3 ± 0.8	8.9 ± 1.1

[a] Data are shown as mean ± S.E.

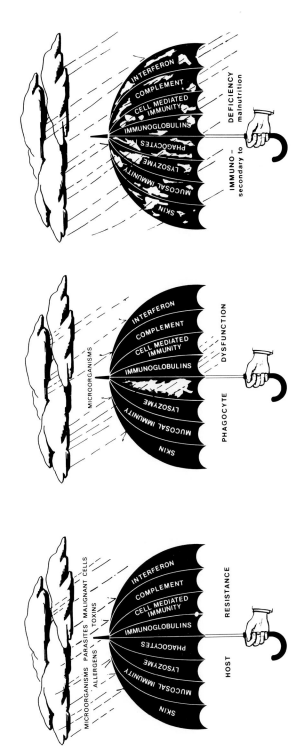

FIG. 1. Host protective factors and examples of primary and secondary immunodeficiency. A concert of nonspecific barriers and antigen-specific immune responses protects man from extraneous and internal injurious agents (*left panel*). Primary, often inherited, deficit of a protective mechanism, for example phagocyte defect, results in repeated severe infections (*center panel*). Malnutrition robs the host of many host defenses (*right panel*). Some bulwarks of immunity are impaired more often and to a greater extent than others. (From ref. 25.)

TABLE 3. Pneumocystis carinii *infection in acute lymphoblastic leukemia*

Group	Serum albumin (g/dl)	Serum transferrin (mg/dl)
Infected	2.7 ± 0.4[a]	121 ± 29
Noninfected	3.4 ± 0.3	198 ± 23

[a] Data are expressed as mean ± S.E.

2. Concurrent or recent infections may suppress immunocompetence and further increase nutritional deficiency. An example is measles which is associated with cutaneous anergy for several weeks, impaired lymphocyte response to mitogens such as phytohemagglutinin (Fig. 2), normal or slightly reduced proportion of rosette-forming T cells, and frequent reactivation of latent infections such as tuberculosis.

3. Our knowledge of the threshold of severity of immunologic dysfunction which is clinically relevant is limited. How much reduction in T cells is biologically important? We do know that complement C3 concentration must fall to less than 40% of control values before it impairs opsonization. On the other hand, a coexistent deficit in antibody response may compound the immunologic problem; now, even a milder impairment of complement system may affect opsonization.

4. Different causes of nutrient deficiency may have different effects on immunity. For example, iron deficiency due to blood loss has relatively little effect on immunocompetence, whereas iron deficiency due to reduced dietary intake does.

5. The many variables of the study design should be similar before comparisons can be valid. This includes the nature and dose of antigen, duration of culture, etc.

6. Results obtained in experiments *in vitro* may have little relevance to findings *in vivo*.

7. The extrapolation of results of studies from one species to another is fraught with danger.

TABLE 4. *Postoperative complications*

Preoperative nutritional status	Sepsis (%)	Mortality (%)
Normal	1.7	0.4
Malnourished	6.8	2.3

TABLE 5. *Organisms commonly isolated from patients with PEM*

Group	Organism
Bacteria	*Klebsiella, Pseudomonas, Proteus, Staphylococcus, Mycobacterium*
Viruses	Measles, herpes simplex
Fungi	*Candida, Aspergillus*
Parasites	*Pneumocystis carinii, Giardia lamblia*

LYMPHOID TISSUES

The association of starvation and profound involution of the thymus to the extent that it may be difficult to locate the organ was described well over a century ago. This led to the term "nutritional thymectomy," a finding dramatically observed in animal models of PEM (8). The thymus of undernourished children is usually small on X-ray examination. In patients with kwashiorkor or marasmus, the thymus, on average, weighs less than one-third of the normal organ. Histologic studies of PEM have shown a significant lymphocyte depletion of lymphoid organs (Figs. 3,4). In the thymus, the clear distinction between the densely packed cortex and sparse medulla is ill-defined and Hassal corpuscles appear degenerated, enlarged, and crowded together. This appearance is distinct from that of the thymus in primary defects of the immune system in which the epithelial components also may be absent or less prominent. The histomorphologic changes in the thymus are most marked in those patients who show lymphopenia before death. In the spleen, the periarteriolar cuff of lymphocytes is less prominent. In the lymph node, germinal centers are scanty and small. There is a reduction in the number of small lymphocytes as well as plasma cells.

IMMUNOCOMPETENCE

A number of immunity functions are deranged in PEM (22,30,39,60). The pattern of infections encountered in patients (52) and the marked histologic changes in the thymus in PEM (58) suggest that cell-mediated immunity (CMI) is impaired. This is a consistent observation and is reflected in changes in skin reactions, lymphocyte subpopulations, and *in vitro* responses. Other immune responses altered in PEM include antibody affinity, complement system, mucosal secretory antibody, phagocytes, and lysozyme (Fig. 1).

DELAYED HYPERSENSITIVITY

Cutaneous tests using ubiquitous recall antigens, such as candidin, trichophytin, streptokinase-streptodornase, mumps, and purified protein derivative of tuberculin, evaluate the memory response dependent on T lymphocytes and

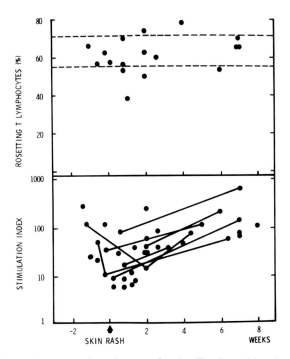

FIG. 2. Effect of measles on number of rosette-forming T cells and lymphocyte proliferation response to phytohemagglutinin. (From ref. 30.)

inflammatory cells and are generally depressed in patients with protein-energy malnutrition (7,23). A direct correlation between the size of induration and concentrations of serum albumin and transferrin has been reported. Skin responses may be impaired in mild to moderate undernutrition. Many studies have also demonstrated marked impairment of the primary afferent or sensitization limb of delayed hypersensitivity, using agents such as keyhole limpet hemocyanin, BCG vaccine, and 2,4 dinitrochlorobenzene (9,45,50,57). Tuberculin conversion after BCG vaccination is impaired and the extent of defect correlates with nutritional status (Table 6).

LYMPHOCYTE SUBPOPULATIONS AND PROLIFERATION RESPONSES

Lymphopenia is seen in approximately 15% of malnourished children; it may be mild or profound. PEM is associated with a reduction in the proportion and absolute number of circulating thymus-dependent T lymphocytes identified by their ability to form rosettes with sheep red blood cells (Fig. 5; refs. 2,11,19,51). Severe malnutrition generally produces a more marked reduction in T-cell number. The mechanism(s) underlying this observation are not clear. Changes in surface membrane proteins including the putative receptor(s) for

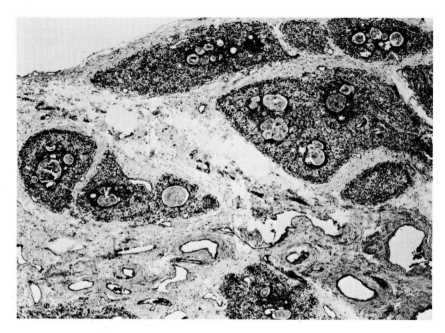

FIG. 3. Thymus in malnutrition. There is a loss of corticomedullary differentiation, fewer lymphoid cells, and degeneration of Hassal bodies. (×25.) (From ref. 39.)

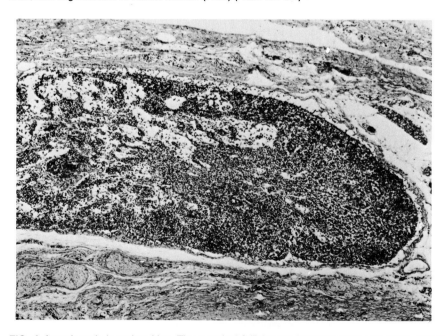

FIG. 4. Lymph node in malnutrition. The germinal follicles are inconspicuous and small. (×25.) (From ref. 39.)

TABLE 6. *Tuberculin conversion 3 months after BCG vaccination*

Nutritional status at time of vaccination	Conversion rate (%)
Normal	82
Mild PEM	68
Moderate PEM	54
Severe PEM	32

sheep red blood cells or the presence of serum inhibitors (3), such as C-reactive protein, IgE, microbial products, and alpha-fetoprotein, can prevent rosette formation with sheep red blood cells, lympholysis due to elevated levels of free cortisol, impaired maturation and differentiation of T-cell precursors, reduction in pre-T cells due to impaired cellular multiplication, and a redistribution of cells to sequestered sites.

Various subsets of T lymphocytes can be distinguished on the basis of cell surface antigens using monoclonal antibodies. These are functionally heterogeneous as well. Our recent studies using monoclonal antibodies and cell sorting technique have demonstrated changes in T-cell subsets in PEM. There is a marked numerical and functional deficiency of T4+ helper cells, whereas T8+ cytotoxic/suppressor cells are affected to a lesser extent (37). These changes in functionally distinct T-lymphocyte subpopulations may explain the alterations in CMI in children with PEM.

The proportion and absolute number of B lymphocytes are similar in well nourished and PEM subjects (2,19), although the latter have a slightly higher

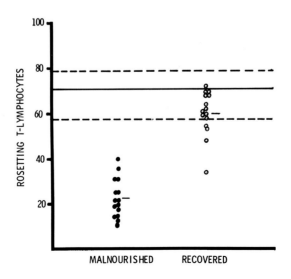

FIG. 5. Rosette-forming T cells in malnutrition and after nutritional rehabilitation.

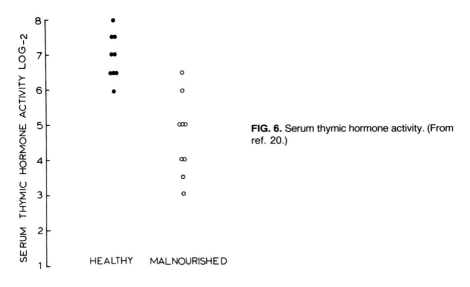

FIG. 6. Serum thymic hormone activity. (From ref. 20.)

proportion of B_α cells (21). Thus, the proportion of "null" cells without the conventional surface markers of T and B lymphocytes is markedly increased. The possibility that these cells may be undifferentiated T lymphocytes is suggested by a significant decrease in serum thymic hormone activity in infants and young children with PEM (Fig. 6; ref. 20) and an elevation in leukocyte terminal deoxynucleotidyl transferase (21). The addition of calf thymic extract *in vitro* to mononuclear cell preparations from undernourished individuals results in an increase in the number of rosetting cells.

Lymphocytes obtained from children with PEM respond poorly to mitogens, particularly when cell cultures are set up in autologous sera (3). Plasma of malnourished, often infected, patients contains inhibitory factors and/or may also lack essential supporting factors for cell proliferation. It is essential to use standard methods and plot dose-response curves since optimal concentrations of mitogen to produce maximum stimulation may vary for different cell preparations. The reduction in lymphocyte transformation response in malnutrition correlates with a decrease in the number of rosetting T lymphocytes.

IMMUNOGLOBULIN-ANTIBODY SYSTEM

Hypergammaglobulinemia is a common finding in malnutrition. This may be the result of frequent associated infections as well as reduction in T-suppressor-cell activity. The concentrations of serum immunoglobulins are generally elevated or within the normal range in PEM (22). Associated bacterial and viral infections and parasitic diseases are important determinants of changes in serum immunoglobulin levels, particularly elevated IgA. Plasma half-life of IgG is reduced in these patients (22). In the occasional malnourished child with concomitant or recent infection, serum IgG, and sometimes IgM

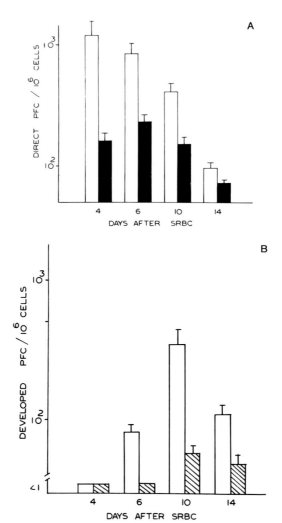

FIG. 7. IgG antibody-forming cells in the spleen of the F_1 generation progeny of starved (*closed or hatched columns*) and control (*open columns*) rats. Three-week-old rats were subjected to partial starvation for 6 weeks. One batch from each experimental and control group was immunized and the animals were killed after 4, 6, 10, or 14 days. Another batch of female rats from the starved and control groups was mated with healthy male animals. On weaning, the litter (F_1 generation) was given free access to food for 6 weeks. These animals were immunized with SRBC and studied for number of direct (IgM) (**A**) and indirect (IgG) (**B**) plaque-forming cells (PFC) in the spleen. Mean and SE are shown, based on data from ref. 14. Copyright 1975, American Association for Advancement of Science.

and IgA, may be low (9). In this situation, plasma half-life of IgG is prolonged (20). Serum IgE concentration is often elevated as a probable result of parasite infection and reduced T-suppressor-cell number and function.

Antibody response is regulated by a number of factors, including the number and function of B and T lymphocytes and macrophages, the dose and nature of the antigen, presence of adjuvant, previous exposure, presence of associated infection, and state of the local lymphoid tissue. Serum antibody response is generally adequate in PEM (9,30,50). Some T-cell-dependent antigens may not induce antibody response to the same extent in PEM as in the healthy state. For example, in nutritionally deprived rats and their offspring, spleen antibody-forming cell response to immunization with sheep red blood cells is reduced (Figs. 7A and 7B; ref. 14).

Secretory IgA

The concentration of secretory IgA and mucosal antibody responses are decreased in moderate to severe PEM (12,53,59). Nasopharyngeal and salivary secretions and tears of malnourished individuals show a reduction in secretory IgA relative to total protein and albumin content. Secretory IgA-antibody response to live attenuated measles and poliovirus vaccines is reduced in malnourished children (12). Antibody is detected less frequently, the time of its first appearance is delayed, the maximum level is significantly lower (Fig. 8). The impairment of the secretory immune system may have several possible consequences. It may contribute to more prolonged and severe illness. It may also permit systemic spread, explaining, in part, the frequent occurrence of gram-negative septicemia in malnutrition. The absorption of macromolecules is increased (13), the clinical significance of which is not clear.

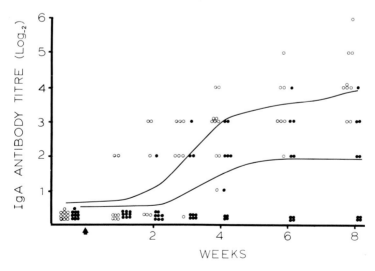

FIG. 8. Secretory IgA-antibody response to live attenuated poliovirus vaccine (*arrow*) in malnourished (*closed circle*) and control (*open circle*) children. (From ref. 12.)

Antibody Affinity

The effect of diet on antibody affinity has been investigated in genetically inbred high- and low-affinity mice (54). Protein deficiency decreased the relative affinity of antibody to human serum albumin in animals normally producing high-affinity antibody. Affinity was not further reduced by protein deprivation of the low-affinity mice.

Complement System

Serum concentrations of almost all complement components are reduced in PEM (18,44). The levels of C4, C5, and C1 inactivator are often within the normal range. Acute starvation and anorexia nervosa also depress C3 levels. In moderate degrees of energy-protein undernutrition, levels of complement component C3 correlate with the extent of weight deficit and biochemical indices of malnutrition as well as with days of febrile illness. Samples from some patients show anticomplementary activity which may be the result of the action of endotoxin, other microbial products, or antigen-antibody complexes. Infection superimposed on malnutrition further depresses the complement system, in contrast to the findings in well nourished subjects in whom complement levels rise in the presence of infection. Degradation products of C3 indicative of consumption are often detected. This, together with reduced hepatic synthesis, may be responsible for the marked reduction in serum C3 concentration seen in nutritional deficiency. The alternate pathway is also altered in PEM. The total activity as well as levels of factor B are decreased (20,44).

Polymorphonuclear Leukocytes

Malnourished children show a slight delay and reduction in the mobilization of monocytes in traumatic Rebuck skin windows and in response to BCG (6). Chemotaxis of polymorphonuclear leucocytes (PMN) initially may be slightly sluggish *in vitro* but, given enough time, the number of cells traversing the barrier are comparable in well nourished and PEM groups, unless infection is present (29). The cellular component of ingestion of opsonized material is adequate, but PMN show several deficits in postphagocytic metabolic burst of oxidative and glycolytic activity. The intracellular killing of ingested bacteria is variably reduced (55,56).

Other Nonspecific Mechanisms

Lysozyme is decreased in the serum and secretions of children with PEM (20,59). Endogenous pyrogen production is decreased. Data on interferon production are inconsistent; some studies have shown a reduction in interferon release from virus-infected leukocytes of PEM patients, others have found a normal response. It is probable that differences in the subjects studied and assay techniques may be important determinants of the different results obtained. Tissue changes may contribute to inadequate physical barriers to the entry of pathogens and may allow easier spread of infection in patients with PEM. These and other nonspecific mechanisms of host defense have been reviewed (20,30,39).

FETAL MALNUTRITION

In developing countries, small-for-gestational-age (SGA) low-birth-weight infants constitute 9 to 30% of all neonates. Infection among these infants is a common cause of morbidity and mortality. Malnutrition occurring during fetal life may be expected to have a more profound and longer-lasting effect on the immune system than acquired postnatal malnutrition. Many studies have indicated that fetal growth retardation is associated with involution of the thymus and impaired CMI (15,33,49). The number of circulating T cells is reduced (Fig. 9) and lymphocyte transformation response to mitogens is decreased. Serum levels of IgG, especially IgG_1 and IgG_3, and antibody titers are lower as a result of decreased placental transfer of immunoglobulins (Fig. 10; ref. 16). Serum concentrations of C3 are decreased and opsonization is suboptimal. The levels of factor B are reduced and correlate with opsonic activity (33). The depression of cell-mediated immunocompetence in SGA low-birth-weight infants has been shown to persist for several months to years (24,31,41,42). In contrast, appropriate-for-gestational-age (AGA) infants of comparable weight recovered their CMI function by the age of 3 months (24). The profound effect of fetal growth retardation on thymic hormone activity

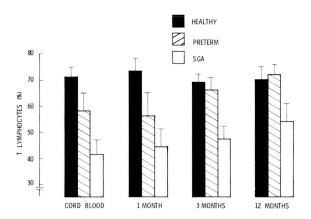

FIG. 9. Rosette-forming T lymphocytes in healthy, preterm appropriate-for-gestational-age, and small-for-gestational-age (SGA) infants. Values shown are means ± SD. (From ref. 24.)

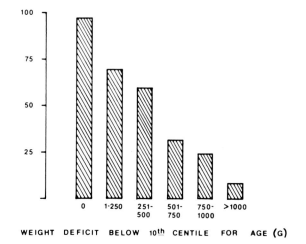

FIG. 10. Percentage distribution of cord tetanus antitoxin levels above the arbitrary protective titer of 0.01 units/ml in infants of mothers immunized during the second trimester of pregnancy. (From ref. 16.)

has been reported recently (24). One-month-old SGA infants show a marked decrease in thymic hormone activity, whereas AGA infants of comparable birth weight have titers that are near normal. These differences in thymic hormone activity in the two groups of low-birth-weight infants appear to provide a prognostic marker, since SGA infants with low thymic hormone activity continue to demonstrate depressed CMI, whereas AGA infants with near normal thymic hormone activity recover immunologically by the age of 3 months. These effects may have clinical and biological significance, particularly frequency, severity, and duration of infection.

DEFICIENCIES OF SINGLE NUTRIENTS

The effects of the deficiencies of individual nutrients have been the subject of much recent work and have been reviewed elsewhere (4,22,27,28,38).

Zinc Deficiency

Zinc deficiency is associated with marked changes in CMI. The lymphoid tissues are atrophic with preferential cellular depletion of the cortex of the thymus and thymus-dependent areas in other organs such as the spleen. Lymphopenia may be observed in a proportion of zinc-deficient subjects. Both primary and secondary antibody responses to T-dependent antigens are reduced (34,43). Recent work indicates that B-cell response to a T-cell-independent antigen, dextran, is also impaired. Delayed cutaneous hypersensitivity is impaired. Zinc-deficient patients and laboratory animals have poor lymphocyte proliferation response to mitogens, and wound healing is impaired.

Mice deprived of zinc for a few weeks show reduction in T-cell cytotoxicity against sensitizing tumor cell targets, particularly *in vivo*, whereas antibody-dependent cell-mediated cytotoxicity is not altered. Recently, Bach (1) has presented evidence for zinc dependency of thymic hormones. Zinc deficiency is associated with decreased levels of thymic hormone (35). The serum thymic factor loses its biological activity after treatment with a metal-chelating agent and the function is restored by the addition of zinc. Many mechanisms may explain the interactions between zinc and the immune system. Zinc is essential for the activity of more than 100 metalloenzymes including thymidine kinase and DNA-dependent RNA polymerase. Zinc stabilizes cell membrane acting at the cytoskeletal level. It can also act as a polyclonal lymphocyte mitogen.

Iron Deficiency

Iron deficiency is prevalent world-wide in all age groups, including infants especially of low birth weight, women in the child-bearing age, elderly and socioeconomically disadvantaged persons. It is important to recognize that iron deficiency can affect multiple systems even prior to a drop in hemoglobin concentration. There are subtle but definite changes in cell-mediated immune responses including T-cell number, *in vitro* lymphocyte proliferation in the presence of mitogens, lymphokine production, and reduced bactericidal capacity of PMN (5,10,17,28,32,46,48). Iron deficiency results in reduced activity of ribonucleotide reductase necessary for DNA synthesis and of myeloperoxidase and hydroxyl radical production. Iron also interacts with many other trace elements which may have important effects on the immune system.

Copper Deficiency

Copper deficiency reduces antibody response to T-cell-dependent antigens, produces neutropenia, and impairs reticuloendothelial function. There is a reduction in T-cell cytotoxicity and in concanavalin A stimulation of lymphocytes. It should be emphasized that there are marked differences between various species with regard to the effects of copper deficiency; thus it is very hazardous to extrapolate such laboratory data to man.

Selenium Deficiency

Selenium has important interactions with vitamin E. Deficiency in both these nutrients reduces antibody responses and changes in hydrogen peroxide levels.

Magnesium Deficiency

Magnesium deficiency in rats results in thymic atrophy in some animals, and thymic hyperplasia and lymphoid malignancy in others.

Vitamin A Deficiency

Vitamin A deficiency reduces lymphocyte proliferation response to mitogens and cell homing patterns, and has significant effects on the complement system.

Pyridoxine Deficiency

Pyridoxine deficiency reduces antibody responses to heterologous red cells, impairs cytotoxicity, decreases serum thymic hormone levels, and impairs lymphocyte proliferation (35,36).

Folic Acid Deficiency

Folic acid deficiency decreases lymphocyte proliferation response to mitogens (40).

Vitamin C Deficiency

Extreme deficiency of vitamin C can impair complement activity and phagocyte function.

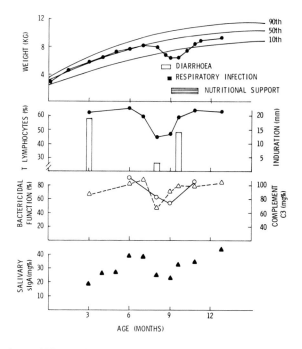

FIG. 11. Growth, morbidity, and immunocompetence assessed periodically in a prospective longitudinal study of an infant. Impaired immune responses were noted earlier than growth failure and preceded clinical evidence of respiratory infection and diarrhea. (From ref. 26.)

Polyunsaturated Fatty Acids

Animals deprived of polyunsaturated fatty acids show reduced antibody responses, both primary and secondary, to several antigens. Cell-mediated immune responses are decreased.

FINAL COMMENTS

Malnutrition and deficits of single nutrients are the most frequent cause of immunodeficiency world-wide (60). The main effects of nutritional imbalance, deficiency and excess, on the immune system have been reviewed above. The influence of moderate PEM on immunocompetence (25,47,61), the rapidity with which immunologic tests show improvement following nutritional therapy of PEM (30), and findings from prospective longitudinal assessment of immunocompetence, growth, and morbidity have led to the suggestion that immunocompetence can be used as a functional index of nutritional status (Fig. 11; ref. 26). These observations should form the basis of multifaceted programs to reduce the intertwined problems of malnutrition and infection (22). It would be desirable to tackle both infection and undernutrition simultaneously.

REFERENCES

1. Bach, J. F. (1981): The multifaceted zinc dependency of the immune system. *Immunol. Today*, 2:225–228.
2. Bang, B. D., Mahalanabis, D., Mukherjee, K. L., and Bang, F. B. (1975): T and B lymphocyte rosetting in undernourished children. *Proc. Soc. Exp. Biol. Med.*, 149:199–202.
3. Beatty, D. W., and Dowdle, E. B. (1979): Deficiency in kwashiorkor serum of factors required for optimal lymphocyte transformation *in vitro. Clin. Exp. Immunol.*, 35:433–437.
4. Beisel, W. R., Edelman, R., Nauss, K., and Suskind, R. M. (1981): Single nutrient effects on immunologic functions. *JAMA*, 245:53–58.
5. Bhaskaram, C., and Reddy, V. (1975): Cell-mediated immunity in iron- and vitamin deficient children. *Br. Med. J.*, 3:522.
6. Bhuyan, U. N., and Ramalingaswami, V. (1974): Systemic macrophage mobilization and granulomatous response to BCG in the protein-deficient rabbit. *Am. J. Pathol.*, 76:313–321.
7. Bistrian, B. R., Blackburn, G. L., Scrimshaw, N. S., and Flatt, J. P. (1975): Cellular immunity in semistarved states in hospitalized adults. *Am. J. Clin. Nutr.*, 28:1148–1153.
8. Borysenko, M., and Lewis, S. (1979): The effect of malnutrition on immunocompetence and whole body resistance to infection in *Chelydra serpentina. Dev. Comp. Immunol.*, 3:89–100.
9. Chandra, R. K. (1972): Immunocompetence in undernutrition. *J. Pediatr.*, 81:1194–1200.
10. Chandra, R. K. (1973): Reduced bactericidal capacity of polymorphs in iron deficiency. *Arch. Dis. Child.*, 48:864–866.
11. Chandra, R. K. (1974): Rosette-forming T lymphocytes and cell-mediated immunity in malnutrition. *Br. Med. J.*, 3:608–609.
12. Chandra, R. K. (1975): Reduced secretory antibody response to live attenuated measles and poliovirus vaccines in malnourished children. *Br. Med. J.*, 2:583–585.
13. Chandra, R. K. (1975): Food antibodies in malnutrition. *Arch. Dis. Child.*, 50:532–535.
14. Chandra, R. K. (1975): Antibody formation in first and second generation offspring of nutritionally deprived rats. *Science*, 190:289–290.
15. Chandra, R. K. (1975): Fetal malnutrition and postnatal immunocompetence. *Am. J. Dis. Child.*, 129:450–455.
16. Chandra, R. K. (1975): Levels of IgG subclasses, IgA, IgM and tetanus antitoxin in paired

maternal and foetal sera. Findings in healthy pregnancy and placental insufficiency. In: *Ma-terno-foetal Transmission of Immunoglobulins*, edited by W. A. Hemmings, pp. 77–90. Cambridge University Press, London.

17. Chandra, R. K. (1975): Impaired immunocompetence associated with iron deficiency. *J. Pediatr.*, 86:899–901.
18. Chandra, R. K. (1975): Serum complement and immunoconglutinin in malnutrition. *Arch. Dis. Child.*, 50:225–228.
19. Chandra, R. K. (1977): Lymphocyte subpopulations in malnutrition: Cytotoxic and suppressor cells. *Pediatrics*, 59:423–428.
20. Chandra, R. K. (1979): Serum thymic hormone activity in protein-energy malnutrition. *Clin. Exp. Immunol.*, 38:228–230.
21. Chandra, R. K. (1979): T and B lymphocyte subpopulations and leukocyte terminal deoxy-nucleotidyl transferase in energy-protein malnutrition. *Acta Paediatr. Scand.*, 68:841–845.
22. Chandra, R. K. (1980): *Immunology of Nutritional Disorders*. Arnold, London.
23. Chandra, R. K. (1980): Cell-mediated immunity in nutritional imbalance. *Fed. Proc.*, 39:3086–3092.
24. Chandra, R. K. (1981): Serum thymic hormone activity and cell-mediated immunity in healthy neonates, preterm infants and small-for-gestational age infants. *Pediatrics*, 67:407–411.
25. Chandra, R. K. (1981): Immunodeficiency in undernutrition and overnutrition. *Nutr. Rev.*, 39:225–231.
26. Chandra, R. K. (1981): Immunocompetence is a functional index of nutritional status. *Br. Med. Bull.*, 37:89–95.
27. Chandra, R. K. (1983): Trace elements and immune responses. *Immunol. Today (in press)*.
28. Chandra, R. K. (1983): *Trace Elements, Immunity and Infection*. Wiley, New York *(in press)*.
29. Chandra, R. K., Chandra, S., and Ghai, O. P. (1976): Chemotaxis, random mobility and mobilization of polymorphonuclear leukocytes in malnutrition. *J. Clin. Pathol.*, 29:224–228.
30. Chandra, R. K., and Newberne, P. M. (1977): *Nutrition, Immunity and Infection: Mechanisms of Interaction*. Plenum, New York.
31. Chandra, R. K., Ali, S. K., Kutty, K. M., and Chandra, S. (1977): Thymus-dependent T lymphocytes and delayed hypersensitivity in low birth weight infants. *Biol. Neonate*, 31:15–18.
32. Chandra, R. K., Au, B., Woodford, G., and Hyam, P. (1977): Iron status, immunocompetence, and susceptibility to infection. In: *Iron Metabolism. Ciba Foundation Symposium No. 51*. Elsevier, Amsterdam.
33. Chandra, R. K., and Matsumura, T. (1979): Ontogenetic development of immune system and effects of fetal growth retardation. *J. Perinat. Med.*, 7:279–287.
34. Chandra, R. K., and Au, B. (1980): Single nutrient deficiency and cell-mediated immune responses. I. Zinc. *Am. J. Clin. Nutr.*, 33:736–738.
35. Chandra, R. K., Au, B., and Heresi, G. (1980): Serum thymic hormone activity in deficiencies of calories, zinc, vitamin A and pyridoxine. *Clin. Exp. Immunol.*, 42:332–336.
36. Chandra, R. K., Au, B., and Heresi, G. (1981): Single nutrient deficiency and cell-mediated immune responses. II. Pyridoxine. *Nutr. Res.*, 1:101–106.
37. Chandra, R. K., Gupta, S., and Singh, H. (1982): Inducer and suppressor T cell subsets in protein-energy malnutrition. Analysis by monoclonal antibodies. *Nutr. Res.*, 2:21–26.
38. Chandra, R. K., and Dayton, D. (1982): Trace element regulation of immunity and infection. *Nutr. Res.*, 2:721–733.
39. Chandra, R. K. (1982): Malnutrition. In: *Primary and Secondary Immunodeficiency Disorders*, edited by R. K. Chandra. Churchill Livingstone, Edinburgh.
40. Coovadia, H. M., Parent, M. A. Loening, W. E., Wesley, A., Burgess, B., Hallett, F., Brian, P., Grace, J., Naidoo, J., Smythe, P. M., and Vos, G.H. (1974): An evaluation of factors associated with the depression of immunity in malnutrition and in measles. *Am. J. Clin. Nutr.*, 27:665–669.
41. Dutz, W., Rossipal, E., Ghavami, H., Vessel, K., Kohout, E., and Post, G. (1976): Persistent cell mediated immune deficiency following infantile stress during the first 6 months of life. *Eur. J. Pediatr.*, 122:117–129.
42. Ferguson, A. C. (1978): Prolonged impairment of cellular immunity in children with intra-uterine growth retardation. *J. Pediatr.*, 93:52–55.

43. Fraker, P. J., Depasquale-Jardieu, P., Zwickle, C. M., and Leucke, R. W. (1978): Regeneration of T-cell helper function in zinc-deficient adult mice. *Proc. Natl. Acad. Sci. USA*, 75:5660–5663.
44. Haller, L., Zubler, R. H., and Lambert, P. H. (1978): Plasma levels of complement components and complement haemolytic activity in protein-energy malnutrition. *Clin. Exp. Immunol.*, 34:248–252.
45. Harland, P. S. (1965): Tuberculin reactions in malnourished children. *Lancet*, i:719–721.
46. Joynson, D. H. M., Jacobs, A., Walker, D. M., and Dolby, A. E. (1972): Defect of cell-mediated immunity in patients with iron-deficiency anemia. *Lancet*, ii:1058–1059.
47. Kielmann, A. A., Uberoi, I. S., Chandra, R. K., and Mehra, V. L. (1976): The effect of nutritional status on immune capacity and immune responses in preschool children in a rural community in India. *Bull. WHO*, 54:477–483.
48. MacDougall, L. G., Anderson, R., McNab, G. M., and Katz, J. (1975): Immune response in iron-deficient children: Impaired cellular defense mechanisms with altered humoral components. *J. Pediatr.*, 86:833–841.
49. Moscatelli, P., Bricarelli, F. G., Piccinini, A., Tomatis, C., and Dufour, M. A. (1976): Defective immunocompetence in foetal undernutrition. *Helv. Paediatr. Acta*, 31:241–247.
50. Neumann, C. G., Lawlor, G. J., Jr., Stiehm, E. R., Swenseid, M. E., Newton, C., Herbert, J., Ammann, A. J., and Jacob, M. (1975): Immunologic responses in malnourished children. *Am. J. Clin. Nutr.*, 28:89–101.
51. Puri, V., Misra, P. K., Saxena, K. C., Saxena, P. N., Saxena, R. P., and Agarwal, C. G. (1980): Immune status in malnutrition. *Indian Pediatr.*, 17:127–132.
52. Purtilo, D. T., and Connor, D. H. (1975): Fatal infections in protein-calorie malnourished children with thymolymphatic atrophy. *Arch. Dis. Child.*, 50:149.
53. Reddy, V., Raghuramulu, N., and Bhaskaram, C. (1976): Secretory IgA in protein-calorie malnutrition. *Arch. Dis. Child.*, 51:871–887.
54. Reinhardt, M. C., and Steward, M. W. (1979): Antibody affinity and clearance function studies in high and low affinity mice. The effect of protein deficiency. *Immunology*, 38:735–739.
55. Selvaraj, R. J., and Bhat, K. S. (1972): Metabolic and bactericidal activities of leukocytes in protein-calorie malnutrition. *Am. J. Clin. Nutr.*, 25:166–172.
56. Seth, V., and Chandra, R. K. (1972): Opsonic activity, phagocytosis and intracellular bactericidal capacity of polymorphs in undernutrition. *Arch. Dis. Child.*, 47:282–284.
57. Sinha, D. P., and Bang, F. B. (1976): Protein and calorie malnutrition, cell-mediated immunity, and B.C.G. vaccination in children from rural west Bengal. *Lancet*, ii:531–534.
58. Smythe, P. M., Brereton-Stiles, G. G., Grace, H. J., Mafoyane, A., Schonland, M., Coovadia, H. M., Loening, W. E., Parent, M. A., and Vos, G. H. (1971): Thymolymphatic deficiency and depression of cell-mediated immunity in protein-calorie malnutrition. *Lancet*, ii:939–943.
59. Watson, R., Reyes, M. A., and McMurray, D. N. (1978): Influence of malnutrition on the concentration of IgA, lysozyme, amylase, and aminopeptidase in children's tears. *Proc. Soc. Exp. Biol. Med.*, 157:215–218.
60. WHO Scientific Group (1978): *Immunodeficiency.* Technical Report Series, 630.
61. Zeigler, H. D., and Ziegler, P. B. (1975): Depression of tuberculin reaction in mild and moderate protein-calorie malnourished children following BCG vaccination. *Johns Hopkins Med. J.*, 137:59–63.

*Acute Diarrhea: Its Nutritional Consequences
in Children*, edited by J. A. Bellanti.
Nestlé, Vevey/Raven Press, New York © 1983.

MALNUTRITION AND IMMUNOLOGICAL RESPONSE

Immunological Deficiencies Related to Diarrheal Diseases

Frederick T. Koster

Division of Infectious Diseases, Department of Medicine, University of New Mexico, Albuquerque, New Mexico 87131

This chapter examines how immune defects may participate in the nutrition-infection interaction in terms of enteric disease susceptibility. The relationship between diarrhea, malnutrition, and immunological defenses is a complex scheme of interactions. Epidemiological studies (25,40) broadly define a limited number of interactions but have failed to provide specific immunological mechanisms. Isolated interactions have been examined in animal models which, while valuable in defining potential relationship, fail to place in perspective the importance of each interaction in the scheme. This chapter will first examine a small number of field studies that have attempted to relate immunologic defects to diarrheal disease in undernourished ambulatory populations. Second, specific immunologic and nonspecific mucosal defense factors will be identified for their vulnerability in nutritional deficiencies, leading to critical mucosal defense defects. It should be noted that the wealth of information on single nutrient deficiencies and immune function (8), as well as on many other factors besides immune defects, which have the microbial and host potential to increase susceptibility to enteric disease (30), will not be considered here.

NUTRITION-IMMUNITY INTERACTIONS IN FIELD STUDIES OF DIARRHEA

Field and epidemiologic studies suffer from the difficulties of separating the large number of dependent and independent variables that determine worsening nutrition and greater infection rates. Design and interpretation of epidemiologic studies must bear in mind the following:

1. Human malnutrition is almost always accompanied by some degree of infection which will have some impact on the nutritional status being measured. Therefore, clinical studies must consider the "malnutrition-infection complex" as an entity. This is a useful and necessary concept (25,40), but creates certain practical difficulties in assigning causality.

151

2. Human malnutrition is a combination of diverse deficiencies. Precise definitions of study populations are required to allow comparison between different studies.

3. Experimental studies which attempt to examine isolated deficiencies probably include multiple undocumented deficiencies.

4. Infections induce nutritional deficiencies and alter immunological responses, perturbations which usually cannot be separated from impaired immunity resulting from nutritional deprivation alone.

5. Host defense is a web of specific immune and nonspecific mechanisms which must be considered as a network rather than isolated events. No study has or will satisfy all these criteria, yet the accumulated literature does implicate immune incompetence in the malnutrition-diarrhea complex.

Diarrheal Morbidity and Nutrition: Field Studies

The classic Guatemalan studies (16,25) and other prospective studies (20,32,35,45) which have related protein-calorie malnutrition (PCM) to increased diarrheal morbidity and mortality will not be reviewed here. Field studies relating diarrhea and immune factors among mild and moderately malnourished children, however, are as scarce as they are difficult to perform and interpret.

A prospective one-year study of 152 Bangladeshi children attempted to relate diarrheal morbidity to nutritional status and cell-mediated immune (CMI) competence (21). As documented in previous studies, poorer nutrition correlated with anergy to three recall antigens and with failure to develop delayed cutaneous hypersensitivity to dinitrochlorobenzene. A positive correlation of poor nutritional status and increased diarrheal morbidity was found only in children over 3 years of age. In this age group, only the best-nourished cohort had significantly fewer days with diarrhea than the other three nutritional cohorts (Table 1). The lack of correlation in children under 3 years may be due to other confounding variables such as breast-feeding or to the predominance of pathogens unaffected by CMI defenses. When skin-test reactivity at

TABLE 1. *Skin-test reactivity to three antigens and subsequent 6-month diarrheal morbidity in children[a]*

Skin-test status (Jan.)	Anergic	Reactive
No. of children	39	53
Mean % of standard weight for height	86.9	90.3
Diarrhea: Jan.–June		
Mean no. episodes	1.6	1.0
Mean episode length (days)	7.7	4.2
Total days diarrhea	13.1	5.0
% Episodes with fever	25.0	13.0

[a] Mild malnourished children (*n* = 92), aged 3 to 10 years, were used in the study.

the onset of study was correlated with subsequent diarrheal morbidity, anergic children had significantly greater morbidity due to diarrheal disease (Table 1) but not to respiratory disease or undifferentiated fever. In the anergic group, the attack rate of diarrhea was increased by 60%, and mean length of each diarrheal episode was increased by 83%, compared with skin-reactive controls. Anergic children also had twice as many diarrheal episodes accompanied by fever as controls. When the data were adjusted for the effect of nutrition on skin-test reactivity and on diarrheal morbidity, the correlations between anergy and diarrhea remained significant. Thus in this population, one measure of T-cell immunocompetence (skin-test response) was an independent determinant of diarrheal morbidity. Future studies need to relate CMI defects to susceptibility to specific enteric pathogens.

This study suggests that defects in CMI relevant to diarrheal disease susceptibility are due to factors other than undernutrition. In the continual cycle of infectious experience by children with mild to moderate PCM, many infections are followed by prolonged anergy. Bangladeshi children convalescing from measles have an increased incidence of diarrheal episodes, which are more likely to be severe and which increase measles-associated mortality threefold (20). Increased susceptibility to diarrhea following measles may be due to persistent anergy (41) or to mucosal defects manifested as a protein-losing enteropathy (6) or both. The impact on mucosal defenses of repeated episodes of diarrhea is poorly understood, yet probably of great clinical importance.

A relationship between CMI and diarrheal disease among malnourished children is supported by a study of 40 malnourished Australian aboriginal children given transfer factor (TF) after nutritional rehabilitation (19). During the 6-month period after TF injection, TF recipients had significantly fewer gastroenteritis episodes, but not fewer chest infection episodes, compared to randomly allocated placebo-injected controls. There was a trend for better growth in the TF recipients. Although this study is difficult to interpret due to inadequate understanding of transfer factor, the two studies at least suggest that more attention needs to be directed to cell-mediated immune defenses in diarrheal disease.

Mucosal Antibody and Nutrition

Unfortunately, few studies have compared diarrheal morbidity between nutritional cohorts and related this to serum or secretory antibody responses. Serum antibody to typhoid parenteral vaccine in severly malnourished children was diminished to both O and H antigens. Serum agglutinating antibody to parenteral administration of killed *Vibrio cholerae* appeared in only one-half of malnourished infants immunized subcutaneously (15); vibriocidal antibody was not impaired. However, the relevance of these observations is minimal in view of the weak correlation between serum antibody and immunity in typhoid fever (18) and cholera (42).

Malnutrition is accompanied by diminished secretory IgA (sIgA) at mucosal surfaces (11), but the significance of this deficiency for increased susceptibility to mucosal infection is not clear. In PCM, there is a 40% reduction in IgA found in nasal secretions, and the degree of reduction does not correlate with presence of overt infection (11). Following parenteral attenuated live measles vaccination, specific nasopharyngeal sIgA antibody failed to appear in some undernourished children, and in others it was both delayed and in significantly lower titer at all test periods compared with normal controls (10), yet serum titers were not impaired. Half of the same undernourished children immunized orally, once, with attenuated polio vaccine failed to develop detectable specific sIgA antibody in secretions, compared with positive responses in all of the controls. A few malnourished children, but no controls, developed specific IgG antibody in secretions. While the humoral immune response appears to be impaired only in extreme malnutrition, antibody at mucosal surfaces may represent a particular response which is more sensitive to a lesser degree of malnutrition.

The levels of sIgA in PCM are considerably greater than the levels seen in adult-acquired hypogammaglobulinemia, half of whom have undetectable serum and secretory IgA (17). Selective IgA deficiency, usually characterized by serum levels less than 0.05 g/liter (normal is 0.5–3.0 g/liter) (31), may have absent or normal secretory IgA production (5,26). Yet, despite the fact that IgA is usually absent in mucosal secretions, only half of such cases suffer from recurrent mucosal infections. The relationship between a local immunoglobulin defect and associated infection is complex. There appears to be two subsets in adult-acquired hypogammaglobulinemia; those who have recurrent upper and lower respiratory tract infection yet appear free from gastrointestinal disease, and those who have a combination of diarrhea, malabsorption, villous atrophy, intestinal lymphocytic infiltrate, achlorhydria, and nodular lymphoid hyperplasia (17). Many, but not all, of the latter group have heavy *Giardia lamblia* infection, which when treated with metronidazole, leads to resolution of the gut disease (2). Presumably the *Giardia* infestation is directly related to sIgA deficiency, although this has not been clearly demonstrated.

A clue to the lack of correlation between IgA deficiency and enteropathic sequellae may be found in the heterogeneity of immunoglobulin deficiencies. IgA deficiency combined with IgG_2 deficiency was accompanied by pyogenic mucosal infections in all cases, whereas none of the subjects with selective IgA deficiency were infected (31). Selective IgA subclass deficiencies are well known to result in recurrent infections (39). Thus, deficiency of certain IgG subclasses may be synergistic with IgA deficiency in increasing susceptibility to mucosal infection. Alternatively, some patients with selective serum and secretory IgA deficiency exhibit compensatory increases in secretory IgM and lactoferrin (5), which may explain a lack of mucosal infection. It is unlikely that sIgA deficiency by itself is a significant determinant of recurrent enteric infections.

MUCOSAL DEFENSE DEFICIENCIES: LABORATORY STUDIES

The paucity of clinical data implicating mucosal immune defects induced by malnutrition suggests that the mucosal barrier should be reexamined. The immune response at the mucosal surface involves a complex sequence of events, outlined in Figs. 1 and 2. This sequence has been reviewed in detail recently (29). Nutritional deficiencies have potential impact on most of the steps in this sequence.

Development of the Mucosal Immune Response

Figure 1 illustrates the events in mucosal-associated lymphoid tissue during the development of a local antibody response. The first step is antigen absorption either by intestinal epithelial cells or specialized absorptive cells overlying collections of organized lymphoid tissue called Peyer's patches. The impact of malnutrition on this step and the subsequent step (step 2) of antigen processing by macrophage-like cells has not been directly studied. Indirect evidence from a study of severely protein-deprived rats immunized orally with cholera toxin (7) suggested that impaired priming by oral toxin was not due primarily to altered absorption of the toxin antigen. The combination, however, of protein-calorie deprivation and lumenal bacterial overgrowth, which deconjugate bile salts, may result in increased absorption of foreign antigens (43).

Maturation of the priming or initial mucosal immune response in Peyer's patches and mesenteric lymph nodes involves both the differentiation of precursor cells into B-cell lymphoblasts and regulatory T cells, and the expansion of these stimulated clones by cell division (steps 3 and 4). The impact of severe protein deprivation on aspects of the differentiation process has been studied. In the rat model of anticholera toxin immunity, protein deprivation of 2 weeks or more severely impaired the priming response to oral toxin, but even after 2 months of deprivation, a period of dietary protein restitution could completely restore the priming response (7). Even the generation of specific sup-

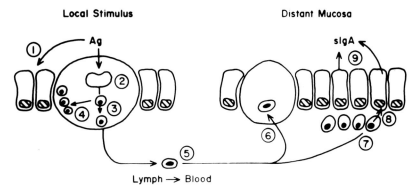

FIG. 1. Schematic drawing of the cellular events of the mucosal antibody response: antigen absorption ① and processing ②, IgA precursor cell differentiation ③ and amplification ④, lymphoblast entry into recirculation from lymph to blood ⑤, lymphocyte homing to Peyer's patches ⑥ and lamina propria ⑦, local secretion of dimeric IgA ⑧, and transport via secretory component through epithelial cells in the gut lumen ⑨.

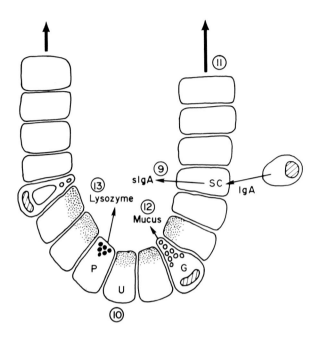

FIG. 2. Schematic drawing of the cellular and secretory immune events in the intestinal crypt epithelium: maturation of undifferentiated cells ⑩ and their migration up the crypt to the villus tip ⑪, the secretion of mucus by goblet cells ⑫, and the secretion of lysozyme by Paneth cells ⑬. U, Undifferentiated (principal) cells; P, Paneth cells; G, goblet cells.

pressor cells in Peyer's patches during the priming response is impaired by protein deprivation, yet dietary protein restitution will completely restore their appearance (34). These studies of mucosal priming suggest that for protein deprivation periods of up to 2 months, cellular differentiation remains intact and protein reconstitution permits amplification of both the B-cell response and T regulator cells.

Following priming events in Peyer's patches and mesenteric lymph nodes, primed lymphoblasts are released into thoracic duct lymph, enter blood, and home preferentially to distant mucosal lymphoid tissue (step 5, Fig. 1). Protein deprivation severely impairs the number of IgA lymphoblasts and specific antitoxin-producing lymphoblasts which enter the lymph after mucosal priming (7). In addition, protein-calorie deprivation and vitamin A deficiency both conspire to impair primed lymphoblasts from preferentially homing to mucosal tissue (27). Thus, amplification and dissemination of priming by means of preferential homing, features unique to the mucosal lymphoid system, are both impaired by deficiencies of protein and other nutrients.

A portion of primed lymphoblasts home to distant Peyer's patches as memory cells (step 6), and some home to gut lamina propria (step 7) where they function as effector cells or memory cells (33). Thus, stimulation of memory cells during a secondary response occurs in both sites and impairment of the secondary response by protein deprivation occurs in both Peyer's patches and lamina propria (34).

It should be noted that in most of the rodent studies discussed above, severe protein deprivation was induced by a diet in which only 4% of calories were derived from protein, compared to 20% in control groups. Such deprivation reduces body weight by 30 to 60% and total lymphoid tissue by 80 to 90% (9), and renders extrapolations to human undernutrition difficult.

Antibody–Nonspecific Factor Interaction at the Mucosa

Until recently, investigations on the impact of malnutrition on mucosal defense have been restricted to considering each mechanism as an isolated entity. Rather, discussion of immunological deficiencies predisposing to diarrhea must include the interaction of multiple deficiencies of mucosal secretory products (3).

Few studies have addressed the question if effector cells reaching mucosal sites are competent to perform their function. Expulsion of *Nippostrongylus brasiliensis* in protein- and iron-deficient rats was studied by adoptively immunizing with transfer of immune lymphocytes to syngeneic infected recipients (14). Immunity was transferred regardless of the nutritional status of the immune donor, yet normal immune lymphocytes transferred to deficient recipients failed to provide immune expulsion. Although it is not clear which deprived nutrient contributed to the deficient immunity, the study does suggest that the deficit was at the final mucosal stage of the response (sites 8 and 9, Fig. 1; and sites in Fig. 2).

Mucus participates in mucosal defense as a lubricant and barrier (site 12, Fig. 2). Among convincing evidence that mucin is important is the observation that certain successful microbes possess strategies to circumvent it; i.e., cholera vibrios produce a mucinase. Mucus release is stimulated by antigen and immune complexes (22). Secretory IgA, which has its own role in the selective immune exclusion of antigens from mucosal surfaces, also nonspecifically increases the affinity of pathogenic salmonellae for mucus (23), thus potentiating nonimmune exclusion.

Goblet cells, the primary factories of intestinal mucin, turn over every 3 days as they migrate out of the crypts and are shed. Protein deficiency markedly impairs epithelial cell renewal (sites 10 and 11, Fig. 2), including goblet cells (13). Induction of isolated vitamin A deficiency rapidly results in a 40% decrease in duodenal goblet cells (37). This reduction is best explained by a diminished rate of goblet cell differentiation, rather than reduced cell division or mucin production.

Secretory IgA, apart from its antigen-binding properties, has synergistic nonspecific effects on the antibacterial mechanisms of at least three substances secreted by mucosal epithelia (site 9, Figs. 1 and 2). Lactoferrin is an abundant iron-binding glycoprotein, secreted by neutrophils and mucosal surfaces, including the intestinal mucosa (36). Since lactoferrin has direct bactericidal effect on mucosal pathogens *Streptococcus mutans* and *V. cholerae* (4), it is a logical participant in mucosal defense. The addition of IgA to lactoferrin potentiates its bacteriostatic effect on *Escherichia coli* (36). The production of transferrin is one of the most severely impaired proteins in kwashiorkor (28); whether the closely related lactoferrin is similarly impaired at mucosal surfaces has not been reported.

Lysozyme, secreted by Paneth cells in intestinal crypts, a variety of mucosal epithelia and neutrophils, has relatively weak bacteriostatic effects (24). Immune bacteriolysis by colostral IgA antibody and complement may (1) require lysozyme. Lysozyme content of saliva from malnourished children is clearly decreased (46); this deficiency coupled with sIgA deficiency could be a significant factor in increased susceptibility at mucosal surfaces.

Lactoperoxidase (LPO) in human saliva and tears and myeloperoxidase produced by human colostral leukocytes provide significant antimicrobial defense mechanisms at certain mucosal sites. LPO catalyzes the oxidation of this cyanate by hydrogen peroxide to hypothiocyanite, which inhibits the growth of gram-positive and gram-negative bacteria *in vivo* and *in vitro* (44). The antimicrobial effect of LPO against *S. mutans* is significantly enhanced by sIgA and myeloma IgA (45). The effect appears to depend on IgA binding to LPO and it has been postulated that such complexing may bring the enzyme into closer association with the bacterial cell membrane and facilitate the entry of hypothiocyanite into the cell (44). Myeloperoxidase production by the polymorphonuclear leukocyte is not impaired in malnutrition (38). However, impairment of mucosal LPO secretion in malnutrition has not been studied.

It is difficult to assign clinical significance to any single factor. Secretory IgA, lysozyme, lactoferrin, complement, lactoperoxidase and leukocytes synergize to provide effective mucosal defense in the absence of specific antibody. It seems reasonable to hypothesize that deficiencies in multiple factors would likewise result in substantial host defects; this hypothesis should be tested.

SUMMARY

The malnutrition-infection complex increases the susceptibility to enteric disease, and immunoincompetence is a logical participant in the cycle of recurrent infections. However, little direct evidence convincingly implicates either CMI defects or secretory IgA deficiency. The lack of clear data on which immune and nonspecific defense mechanisms are critical for protection against specific enteric pathogens makes the investigative task difficult. Future studies correlating nutritional deficiencies and mucosal defense defects in diarrheal disease should take a broader approach to the multiple protective factors in the mucosal barrier.

REFERENCES

1. Adinolfi, M., Glynn, A. A., Lindsay, M., and Milne, C. M. (1966): Serological properties of vA antibodies to *Escherichia coli* present in human colostrum. *Immunology*, 10:517–526.

2. Ament, M. E., and Rubin, C. E. (1972): Relation of giardiasis to abnormal intestinal structure and function in gastrointestinal immunodeficiency syndromes. *Gastroenterology*, 62(2):216–226.
3. Annotations (1979): The interaction of antibacterial factors in breast milk. *Dev. Med. Child. Neurol.*, 21:808–819.
4. Arnold, R. R., Cole, M. F., and McGhee, J. R. (1977): A bactericidal effect for human lactoferrin. *Science*, 5:263–265.
5. Arnold, R. R., Prince, S. J., Mestecky, J., Lynch, D., Lynch, M., and McGee, J. R. (1978): Secretory immunity and immunodeficiency. In: *Secretory Immunity and Infection*, edited by J. R. McGhee, J. Mastecky, and J. L. Babb. pp. 401–410. Plenum Press, New York.
6. Axton, J. H. (1975): Measles: A protein-losing enteropathy. *Br. Med. J.*, 3:79–80.
7. Barry, W. S., and Pierce, N. F. (1979): Protein deprivation causes reversible impairment of mucosal immune response to cholera toxoid/toxin in rat gut. *Nature*, 281(5726):64–65.
8. Beisel, W. R. (1982): Single nutrients and immunity. *Am. J. Clin. Nutr.*, Feb. supplement, 35:417–468.
9. Bell, R. G., Hazell, L. A., and Price, P. (1976): Influence of dietary protein restriction on immune competence II. Effect on lymphoid tissue. *Clin. Exp. Immunol.*, 26:314–326.
10. Chandra, R. K. (1975): Reduced secretory antibody response to live attenuated measles and poliovirus vaccines in malnourished children. *Br. Med. J.*, 2:583–585.
11. Chandra, R. K. (1977): Immunoglobulins and antibody response in protein calorie malnutrition—a review. In: *Malnutrition and the Immune Response*, edited by R. M. Suskind, pp. 155–168. Raven Press, New York.
12. Coovadia, H. M., Parent, M. A., Loening, W. E. K., Wesley, A., Burgess, B., Hallett, F., Brain, P., Grace, J., Naidoo, J., Smythe, P. M., and Vos, G. H. (1974): An evaluation of factors associated with the depression of immunity in malnutrition and in measles. *Am. J. Clin. Nutr.*, 27:665–669.
13. Deo, M. G., and Ramalingaswami, V. (1964): Absorption of Co⁵⁸ labeled cyanocobalamin in protein deficiency. An experimental study in the rheesus monkey. *Gastroenterology*, 46:167–174.
14. Duncombe, V. M., Bolin, T. D., Davis, A. E., and Kelly, J. D. (1981): Delayed expulsion of the nematode Nippostrongylus brasiliensis from rats on a low protein diet: the role of a bone marrow derived component. *Am. J. Clin. Nutr.*, 34:400–403.
15. El-Molla, A., El-Ghoroury, A., Hussein, M., Bodr-el-din, M. K., Hassan, A. H. I., Aref, G. H., and El-Araby, I. (1973): Antibody production in protein calorie malnutrition. *J. Trop. Med. Hyg.*, 76:248–251.
16. Gordon, J. E., Guzman, M. A., Ascoli, W., and Scrimshaw, N. S. (1964): Acute diarrheal disease in less developed countries. 2. Patterns of epidemiological behavior in rural Guatemalan villages. *Bull. WHO*, 31:9–20.
17. Hermans, P. E., Diaz-Buxo, J. A., and Stobo, J. D. (1976): Idiopathic late-onset immunoglobulin deficiency. Clinical observations in 50 patients. *Am. J. Med.*, 61:221–237.
18. Hornick, R. B., Greisman, S. E., Woodward, T. E., DuPont, H. L., Dawkins, A. T., and Snyder, M. J. (1970): Typhoid fever: Pathogenesis and immunologic control. *N. Engl. J. Med.*, 283:739–746.
19. Jose, D. G., Ford, G. W., and Welch, J. S. (1976): Therapy with parents lymphocyte transfer factor in children with infection and malnutrition. *Lancet*, 1:263–266.
20. Koster, F. T., Curlin, G. C., Ariz, K. M. A., and Hague, A. (1982): Synergistic impact of measles and diarrhea on nutrition and mortality in Bangladesh. *Bull. WHO* 59:901–908.
21. Koster, F. T., Palmer, D. L., Chakraborty, J., Shepard, R., Jackson, T., and Curlin, G. C. (1982): Cellular immune competence and diarrheal morbidity in malnourished Bangladeshi children. (*Submitted for publication.*)
22. Lake, A. M., Bloch, K. J., Neutra, M. R., and Walker, W. A. (1979): Intestinal goblet cell mucus release. II. *In vivo* stimulation by antigen in the immunized rat. *J. Immunol.*, 122(3):834–837.
23. Magnusson, K. E., and Stjernstrom, I. (1982): Mucosal barrier mechanisms. Interplay between secretory IgA (SIgA), IgG and mucins on the surface properties and association of salmonellae with intestine and granulocytes. *Immunology*, 45:239–248.
24. Martinez, R. J., and Carroll, S. F. (1980): Sequential metabolic expressions of the lethal process in human serum-treated Esherichia coli: Role of Lysozyme. *Infect. Immun.*, 28(3):735–745.
25. Mata, L. J. (1975): Malnutrition-infection interactions in the tropics. *Am. J. Trop. Med. Hyg.*, 24:564–574.

26. McClelland, D. B. L., Shearman, D. J. C., and Van Furth, R. (1976): Synthesis of immunoglobulin and secretory component by gastrointestinal mucosa in patients with hypogammaglobulinaemia or IgA deficiency. *Clin. Exp. Immunol.*, 25:103–111.

27. McDermott, M. R., Mark, D. A., Befus, A. D., Baliga, B. S., Suskind, R. M., and Bienenstock, J. (1982): Impaired intestinal localization of mesenteric lymphoblasts associated with vitamin A deficiency and protein-calorie malnutrition. *Immunology*, 45:1–5.

28. McFarlane, H., Reddy, S., Adcock, K. J., Adeshina, H., Cooke, A. R., and Akene, J. (1970): Immunity, transferrin and survival in kwashiorkor. *Br. Med. J.*, 4:268–270.

29. Mestecky, J., McGhee, J. R., Crago, S. S., Jackson, S., Kilian, M., Kiyono, H., Babb, J. L., and Michalek, S. M. (1980): Molecular-cellular interactions in the secretory IgA response. *J. Reticuloendothel. Soc.*, 28(Suppl.):45–60.

30. Murray, J. M., and Murray, A. B. (1981): Letter: Paradoxical interrelationships of test of immune function and host resistance in nutritional deficiency—a caution to immunologists. *Am. J. Clin. Nutr.*, 34/6:1159–1160.

31. Oxelius, V. A., Laurell, A. B., Lindquist, B., Golebiowska, H., Axelsson, U., Bjorkander, J., and Hanson, L. A. (1981): IgG subclasses in selective IgA deficiency. Importance of IgG2-IgA deficiency. *N. Engl. J. Med.*, 304(24):1476–1477.

32. Palmer, D. L., Koster, F. T., Alam, A. K. M. J., and Islam, M. R. (1967): Nutritional states: A determinant of severity of diarrhea in patients with cholera. *J. Infect. Dis.*, 134:8–14.

33. Pierce, N. F., and Gowans, J. L. (1975): Cellular kinetics of the intestinal immune response to cholera toxoid in rats. *J. Exp. Med.*, 142:1550–1563.

34. Pierce, N. F., Koster, F. T., and Barry, W. S. (1981): Impairment of the enteric secretory immune response by protein deprivation. In: *Nutritional Factors: Modulating Effects on Metabolic Processes*, edited by R. F. Beers, Jr. and E. G. Bassett, pp. 405–415. Raven Press, New York.

35. Puffer, R. R., and Serrano, C. V. (1973): Patterns of mortality in childhood. *Pan American Health Organization* (Washington, D.C.), Scientific Publication No. 262, p. 146.

36. Rogers, H. J., and Synge, C. (1978): Bacteriostatic effect of human milk on Escherichia coli: The role of IgA. *Immunology*, 34:19–28.

37. Rojanapo, W., Lamb, A. J., and Olson, J. A. (1980): The prevalence, metabolism and migration of goblet cells in rat intestine following the induction of rapid, synchronous vitamin A deficiency. *J. Nutr.*, 110:178–188.

38. Schopfer, K., and Douglas, S. D. (1976): Deutrophil function in children with Kwashiorkor. *J. Lab. Clin. Med.*, 88(3):450–461.

39. Schur, P. H., Borel, H., Gelfand, E. W., Alper, C. A., and Rosen, F. S. (1970): Selective gamma-G globulin deficiencies in patients with recurrent pyogenic infections. *N. Engl. J. Med.*, 283(12):631–634.

40. Scrimshaw, N. S., Taylor, C. E., and Gordon, J. E. (1968): Interactions of nutrition and infection. *World Health Organization* (*Geneva*), Monograph Serial No. 57. 60–142.

41. Shittle, H. C., Dossetor, J., Oduloju, A., Bryceson, A. D. M., and Greenwood, B. M. (1978): Cell-mediated immunity during natural measles infection. *J. Clin. Invest.*, 62:678–84.

42. Svennerholn, A-M. (1980): The nature of protective immunity in cholera. In: *Cholera and Related Diarrheas*, pp. 171–184. 43rd Nobel Symposium, Stockholm.

43. Teichberg, S., Fagundes-Neto, U., Bayne, M. A., and Lifshitz, F. (1981): Jejunal macromolecular absorption and bile salt deconjugation in protein-energy malnourished rats. *Am. J. Clin. Nutr.*, 34:1281–1291.

44. Tenovuo, J., Moldoveanu, Z., Mestecky, J., Pruitt, M., Rahemtulla, B. (1982): Interaction of specific and innate factors of immunity: IgA enhances the antimicrobial effect of the lactoperoxidase system against streptococcus mutans. *J. Immunol.*, 128(2):726–731.

45. Trowbridge, F., and Newton, L. H. (1979): Seasonal changes in malnutrition and diarrheal diseases among preschool children in El Salvador. *Am. J. Trop. Med. Hyg.*, 28:135–141.

46. Watson, R. R., Reyes, M. A., and McMurray, D. N. (1978): Influence of malnutrition on the concentration of IgA, lysozyme, amylase, and Aminopeptidase in children's tears. *Proc. Soc. Exp. Biol. Med.*, 157:215–219.

Acute Diarrhea: Its Nutritional Consequences in Children, edited by J. A. Bellanti.
Nestlé, Vevey/Raven Press, New York © 1983.

Malnutrition and Immunological Response

Diarrhea and Immunity

Rodrigo C. Hurtado

5597 Seminary Road, Baileys Crossroads, Virginia 22041

An excellent review has been presented describing how immune defense mechanisms may participate in nutrition-infection interaction, with special emphasis on the diarrheic syndrome (F. Koster, *this volume*).

The identification of specific and nonspecific immunological and nonimmunological mucosal defense factors has been carefully done. In addition, the concept of a local immune system and its impairment by malnutrition has become widely accepted.

The studies attempting to relate diarrheal morbidity to nutritional status and cell-mediated immunity are significant in correlating anergy and diarrhea (7).

Also, the relationship between cell-mediated immunity and diarrhea, after use of a transfer factor (5), is another piece of evidence for this complex but fascinating interaction.

Adding to the above, it seems that diarrhea after measle infection could be an expression of a depressed cell-mediated immunity leading to this condition (6,12). It has also been suggested that malnutrition is accompanied by diminished secretory IgA at mucosal surfaces (3), although this is not necessarily associated with increased susceptibility to mucosal infections.

Also, the impairment of some unspecific mechanisms, such as lactoferrin and lysozyme in malnutrition (9,14), may contribute to the association malnutrition-diarrhea.

Once the existence of an interaction between immunodepression and diarrhea has been accepted, a reverse question arises. Could the acute diarrheal syndrome cause an immunodeficiency?

The understanding of the regulatory mechanisms of the immune response in the gastrointestinal tract may offer some support to this.

The immune exclusion of feeding antigens or Schulzberger-Chase phenomenon is a function of secretory IgA. Also, secretory IgA coupled antigen enters the portal circulation and is transported by the hepatocyte to the biliary system (2,11,13). The hepatobiliary transport of IgA functions as a mechanism for the removal of macromolecular IgA-complexed antigens, which circumvents the inflammatory consequences of phagocytosis and complement activation.

Environmental orally absorbed antigens induce preferentially activation of T cells in Peyer's patches (4) and result in the generation of IgA class-specific helper T lymphocytes, with subsequent increase of the IgA B-lymphocyte precursor pool and expansion of the IgA memory B-cell pool. At the same time, antigen feeding results in the generation of antigen-specific IgG suppressor T cells in the Peyer's patches (8) preventing unwanted systemic reactions against the absorbed antigen. It can be postulated that terminal differentiation to IgA-producing plasma cells can only occur in tissues where the ratio of class-specific T suppressor to the T helper cells favors the IgA synthesis.

It has also been shown (10) that antigen feeding induces the generation of IgE-specific suppressor T cells in the Peyer's patches, probably similar to the way it happens with IgG. Colostrum feeding is accompanied by the specific regulatory influence of IgE synthesis.

Any changes in this regulatory mechanism may lead to at least a temporary imbalance in the production of different types of antibodies in the mucosal system. The question arises then, if a bowel infection per se could change the regulatory mechanism. Certain viruses or bacteria could locally alter the regulatory mechanism that balances production of IgA-IgG-IgE, perhaps reversing the normal pattern. If this is the case, it could explain why the genesis of local or even systemic manifestations of allergic disorders can be regarded as an expression of an immune imbalance.

REFERENCES

1. Bazin, H., Andre, C., and Heremans, J. F. (1973): Responses immunologiques induites par voie orale. *Ann. Immunol. (Inst. Pasteur),* 124C:253.
2. Birbeck, M. S. C., Cartwright, P., Hall, J. G., Orlans, E., and Peppard, J. (1979): The transport by hepatocytes of immunoglobulin A from blood to bile visualised by autoradiography and electron microscopy. *Immunology,* 37:477.
3. Chandra, R. K. (1977): Immunoglobulins and antibody response in protein calorie malnutrition: a review. In: *Malnutrition and the Immune Response,* edited by R. M. Suskind, pp. 155–168. Raven Press, New York.
4. Gearhart, P., and Cebra, J. J. (1978): Differential expression of IgA by Peyer's patch B cells specific for environmental antigens. *Fed. Proc.,* 37:1396.
5. Jose, D. G., Ford, G. W., and Welch, J. S. (1976): Therapy with parents lymphocyte transfer factor in children with infection and malnutrition. *Lancet,* 1:263–266.
6. Koster, F. T., Curlin, G. C., Aziz, K. M. A., and Hague, A. (1982): Synergistic impact of measles and diarrhea on nutrition and mortality in Bangladesh. *Bull. WHO,* 59:901–908.
7. Koster, F. T., Palmer, D. L., Chakrabory, J., Shepard, R., Jackson, T., and Curlia, G. C. (1982): Cellular immune competence and diarrheal morbidity in malnourished Bangladeshi Children. (*Submitted for publication.*)
8. Mattingly, J. A. (1978): Antigen-specific suppressor T cells formed in the Peyer's patches of rats after oral ingestion of antigen. *Fed. Proc.,* 37:1491.
9. McFarlane, H., Reddy, S., Adcock, K. J., Adeshiar, H., Cooke, A. R., and Akene, J. (1970): Immunity, transferrin and survival in kwashiorkor. *Br. Med. J.,* 4:268–270.
10. Ngan, J., and Kind, L. S. (1978): Suppressor T cells for IgE and IgA in Peyer's patches of mice made tolerant by oral administration of oral serum. *J. Immunol.,* 120:861.
11. Orlans, E., Peppard, J., Reynolds, J., and Hall, J. (1978): Rapid Active transport of immunoglobulin A from blood to bile. *J. Exp. Med.,* 147:588.
12. Shittle, H. C., Dossetor, J., Oduloju, A., Bryceson, A. D. M., and Greenwood, B. M. (1978): Cell mediated immunity during natural measles infection. *J. Clin. Invest.,* 62:678–684.
13. Socken, D. J., Jee Jee Bhoy, K. N., Bazin, H., and Underdown, B. J. (1979): Identification of secretory component as an IgA receptor on rat hepatocytes. *J. Exp. Med.,* 150:1538.
14. Watson, R. R., Reyes, M. A., and McMurray, D. N. (1978): Influence of malnutrition on the concentration of IgA, lysozyme, amylase, and aminopeptidase in children's tears. *Proc. Soc. Exp. Biol. Med.,* 157:215–219.

Acute Diarrhea: Its Nutritional Consequences in Children, edited by J. A. Bellanti.
Nestlé, Vevey/Raven Press, New York © 1983.

MALNUTRITION AND IMMUNOLOGICAL RESPONSE

Discussion

Dr. Edelman: I should like to ask Dr. Chandra whether there is a relationship between antibody affinity and malnutrition. I do not remember him discussing whether there are any changes in the type of antibody that is produced in malnourished individuals.

Dr. Chandra: Studies mostly conducted in mice and rats have shown that both protein deficiency and deficiencies of single amino acids do have an influence on affinity with the result that the handling of subsequently administered antigens is abnormal; there is a greater incidence of immune complex formation with more deposits in the kidney and other sites as a result of those immune complexes. The interesting thing is that in some of these animal studies, the nutrient deficiency was such that it did not cause a change in weight of the animal. In the case of a specific amino acid deficiency such as tryptophan, for example, while the deficiency did not result in weight reduction, it still produced a distinct reduction in antibody affinity.

Dr. Bellanti: One of the effects of severe malnutrition in children is a reduction in size of the thymus. This is a constant finding and has been used by the pathologist as a marker of severe malnutrition. I would add a word of caution, however, concerning the measurement of T-cell sets because, as the technology improves, we are learning that the T-cell population is no longer considered homogeneous: it is probably divisible into three or four subsets.

Acute Diarrhea: Its Nutritional Consequences in Children, edited by J. A. Bellanti.
Nestlé, Vevey/Raven Press, New York © 1983.

ROLE OF BREAST-FEEDING IN THE
NUTRITIONAL STATUS OF INFANTS

Role of Breast-Feeding for the Nutrition and Immunologic Development of the Infant

*R. Lodinová-Žadníková and *†H. Tlaskalova-Hogenova

*Research Institute for the Care of Mother and Child; and †Department of
Immunology, Institute of Microbiology, Czechoslovak Academy
of Science, Prague, Czechoslovakia*

For about 200 million years, mammals have been feeding their babies with their own milk. Humans have been the only species to interrupt the practice by making milk products for artificial feeding. Formulas based on cow's milk became available in many countries, without knowing enough about the consequences of their use.

In the past ten years, new information on human milk has accumulated based on modern scientific research, including biochemistry, nutrition, immunology, endocrinology, and psychophysiology. Human milk is a highly complex and unique secretion quite different from the milk of other species. It contains many constituents which are present in proportions and chemical forms different from those found in milks of other species. We still know very little about many of them, in spite of the hundreds of scientific papers which have been published during the last decade.

NUTRITIONAL COMPONENTS OF BREAST MILK

The composition and output of human milk have been discussed recently in a number of review papers and we shall, therefore, not deal with this aspect of breast-feeding (7,14,33).

IMMUNOLOGIC COMPONENTS OF BREAST MILK

Direct nutritional considerations cannot be viewed in isolation from other related aspects such as host resistance to infections and the consequences of the mother-child relationship. Breast-feeding is much more than the simple supplying of nutrients to the baby. It is a biological interaction of wide importance. Apart from nutritional and metabolic considerations, mammalian milk appears to provide specific protective factors during the time when the newborns are becoming adjusted to the risks of the extrauterine environment. In man, recent evidence suggests that such factors are not only antiinfective, but also help to protect against the early development of some forms of infant allergy. It has also been shown in animal experiments that breast-feeding influences the development of immunologic capacity.

Although the newborn organism is able to respond to different antigens, the response is quantitatively low and also differs qualitatively from that of the adult organism (28). In some species, including man, this disadvantage is compensated by the transfer of humoral antibodies from mother to the offspring via placenta; in other species (pig, sheep) the transfer of immunoglobulins occurs only through the colostrum and milk. Even though the very life of the human infant does not depend on breast-feeding, the protective effect against infection has been clinically recognized for decades (5).

The protective effect of colostrum and milk is multifactorial, including all known types of immunologic mechanisms, i.e., nonspecific, specific, humoral, and cellular. The antibodies received by the human fetus *in utero* act largely against certain systemic infections while resistance factors from the breast-milk appear to act mainly within the intestine.

HUMORAL FACTORS

Various protective factors are present in human milk, including immunoglobulins, lysozyme, the bifidus factor, and nutrient-carried proteins which bind vitamin B_{12}, folate, and iron, and limit their availability to intestinal bacteria, especially *Escherichia coli*.

Milk contains large amounts of lactoferrin, an unsaturated iron-binding compound having a strong antibacterial effect, by limiting the availability of iron for bacterial growth. It has been suggested that lactoferrin acts synergistically with IgA, especially against pathogenic strains of *E. coli* and *Candida albicans*. Because lactoferrin competes for iron with enteral organisms, the use of supplementary iron in breast-fed infants may be contraindicated as interfering with the protection afforded by lactoferrin (3).

The *bifidus factor* in human milk, characterized as a nitrogen-containing polysaccharide, facilitates the growth of *Lactobacillus bifidus*, which appears to have the function of checking the growth of undesirable, possibly harmful, organisms such as enteropathogenic *E. coli*, by producing acetic and lactic acid, thereby lowering the pH of the stool (5).

Lysozyme (muramidase), the well recognized antiinfective substance in lacrymal secretion, is also found in breast-milk in about 5,000 higher concentration than in cow's milk (12). This enzyme causes the lysis of gram-positive and some gram-negative bacteria by hydrolyzing the linkage between muramic acid and N-acetylglucosamine of the bacterial cell wall.

Recently, evidence has been obtained for the presence of all nine components of *complement* in human colostrum. They might be activated through the classic pathway by IgM and IgG antibodies present in low amounts in colostrum and, in addition, by gram-negative bacteria such as *E. coli*. Serum and secretory IgA have been reported to be capable of activating complement, especially when aggregated (2). The high *lipase* activity in human milk has been shown to be related to its antiviral activity, acting against several alphaviruses, flaviviruses, herpes simplex virus, oncoviruses, and others. The antistaphylococcus factor identified by Gyorgy (9) has been found in the free fatty-acid fraction of milk. The precise mechanism of antiviral activity of lipids is still unknown.

Other substances also occur, which may have protective functions, such as interferon, derived from milk lymphocytes, which may have antiviral properties. Although the IgG, IgM, and IgA classes of *immunoglobulins* are present in human milk during the whole period of lactation, the highest concentrations, particularly of IgA and IgM classes, are found in the early colostrum. Ig concentrations decline sharply, 5 to 6 days postpartum, as the amount of milk increases and the process of lactation is fully established (21). The levels of IgA remain higher in the colostrum and milk than in the serum. This fact was explained by the finding that IgA is produced locally by cells present in the milk (13) and by experiments in which the selective concentration of serum IgA by mammary glands was proved (11).

The effect of ingested IgA is restricted because it cannot be absorbed from the infant's gut in large amounts. Milk immunoglobulins are absorbed only for a short period after birth (21). Secretory IgA is more resistant to the action of proteolytic enzymes than serum IgA and is found intact in the feces of the infant (17,32). The newborn organism is not able to produce intestinal secretory IgA during the first weeks after birth. Ingestion of secretory IgA in the breast milk leads to high local concentration at potential sites of entry of pathogenic microorganisms and may protect the neonate's gut from invasion of pathogens (5,25). The presence and concentration of milk antibodies depend on the previous and current experience of the mother. Although secretory IgA does not fix complement, it may possibly prevent bacterial adherence to membranes, agglutinate bacteria, and neutralize bacterial toxins (25). The presence of antibodies in milk, mainly directed against antigens occurring in the gut, and the finding of specific cells committed to react with these antigens supports the idea that the mammary gland is a part of the so-called "common mucosal system" in which the migration of cells originating in the gut to mucosal surfaces at distant sites occurs (19,23).

In our own work, we have studied some of the biological activities of immunoglobulins isolated from pig immune colostrum against *E. coli* 055. We have compared the hemagglutinating, hemolytic, and bactericidal activities of these immunoglobulins in pigs, i.e., in the species where colostrum represents the only source of maternal antibodies and is, therefore, of crucial importance. Although the hemagglutinating activity against lipopolysaccharide-sensitized sheep red cells was present in all three immunoglobulins tested, the hemolytic

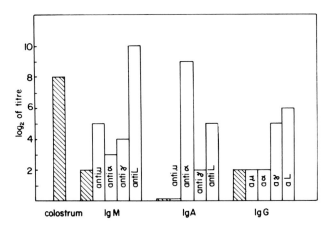

FIG. 1. Hemolytic antibody activity in IgM, IgG, and IgA isolated from the colostrum of pigs immunized with *E. coli* 055 using sheep red blood cells coated with *E. coli* 055 lipopolysaccharide. Initial IgM, IgG, and IgA concentration was 0.2%. Facilitation performed by specific antisera against μ, γ, α, and L chains. *Hatched bar*: direct hemolysis; *clear bar*: indirect hemolysis.

activity was not present in IgA fraction. Using specific antisera for potentiation, we could also detect anti-LPS activity in IgA immunoglobulin (Fig. 1; refs. 27,30). Using bactericidal reaction as a detection system we did not find any inhibitory effect of IgA antibodies with complement on bacterial growth, and we did not succeed in obtaining any bactericidal effect of the mixture consisting of purified IgA and egg-white lysozyme in the presence of complement (Fig. 2). We could, however, demonstrate the beneficial effect of colostral antibodies present in the intestinal tract of germ-free piglets on artificially induced septicemia (Table 1; ref. 29).

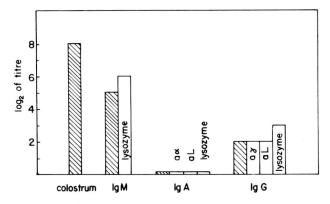

FIG. 2. Bactericidal antibody activity (against *E. coli* 055) in IgM, IgG, and IgA isolated from the colostrum of pigs immunized with *E. coli* 055. Initial IgM, IgG, and IgA concentration was 0.2%. *Hatched bar*: bactericidal reaction; *clear bar*: reaction after adding lysozyme.

TABLE 1. *Effect of immune colostrum and serum[a] on survival of germ-free piglets[b]*

No. of animal	Protein administered	Titer of bactericidal antibodies	Time of death in hr after i.v. contamination
1	Immune colostrum	10^{-12}	Survived
2	Immune colostrum	10^{-12}	14
3	Immune colostrum	10^{-12}	Survived
4	Immune serum	10^{-15}	7
5	Immune serum	10^{-15}	44
6	Immune serum	10^{-15}	Survived
7	Immune serum	10^{-15}	10
8	Immune serum	10^{-15}	Survived
9	—	—	6
10	—	—	8

[a] About 12.5 ml was administered orally 72 hr after birth.
[b] Germ-free piglets were intravenously contaminated with a virulent strain of *Escherichia coli* 055.

Cellular Components

Colostrum and milk contain a large amount of cells which have recently attracted the interest of many workers. Although their fate in the digestive tract of the infant is not fully explained yet, their number, when recalculated in relationship to the amount of milk consumed by the infant, implies that they must play a very important role in the local protection of the intestine. Milk leukocyte counts are in the range of 1 to 3 million/ml. Most cells are of monocytic origin (60–90%) and only about 10% are lymphocytes. The primary cell in human milk appears to be the macrophage. Milk macrophages possess all the typical characteristics such as adherence and spreading on the substrate, high phagocytic activity, alpha-naphtyl esterase positivity, and presence of C3 and Fc receptors. They synthesize lysozyme, complement components, and transferrin. Milk macrophages are more metabolically active than other macrophages, which may be the result of the active phagocytosis of fat particles. The high amount of lactoferrin, components of complement, lysozyme, secretory component, and immunoglobulins of the IgA and IgM classes found in phagocytic cells indicate that they have acquired these proteins by ingestion from the environment. The milk macrophages also release more immunoglobulin than do the lymphocytes, and they may, therefore, serve as a transport vehicle capable of slow, delayed immunoglobulin release (24). Many authors hypothesize that the macrophages are the principal Ig-containing cells in milk and colostrum (6). They can tolerate large variations in the environment and remain active in the milk until digestion, i.e., they may significantly contribute to the defense of the gastrointestinal tract of the infant. Milk lymphocytes are of three main types: T lymphocytes, B lymphocytes, and bearing surface Ig and null cells that cannot be grouped in either the T or B category.

The T lymphocytes respond to antigens that are present in the gut, for example, to K antigens of *E. coli*, but they are unresponsive to others, such as tetanus toxoid or *Candida albicans*. Thus, it seems that the mammary gland is able to select some cells or clones from the repertoire of natural immunologic reactivities by a mechanism similar to that responsible for the local mucosal immunity in the gut (23). Some data suggest that tuberculin-specific cell-mediated immunity can be transferred from the mother to the suckling rat via colostrum and milk. This reactivity can represent an uptake of antigen-sensitized intact cells or mediators released by the maternal T lymphocytes in the intestinal tract of the newborn (10). Clinical studies suggest that a limited number of macromolecules can cross the mucosal barrier even under physiologic conditions in man. In newborns, particularly in premature infants, many of the factors controlling the uptake of intestinal proteins such as secretory IgA, mucoproteins, and adsorbed pancreatic enzymes are undeveloped. This allows for increased access of intestinal antigens to the systemic circulation (31). Many factors in human milk can facilitate the maturation of the intestinal barrier.

Recently, it has been proven in animals that lymphoblasts in gut associated lymphoid tissue come home to the mammary gland and differentiate there into IgA-containing plasmablasts. This phenomenon is limited to lactating recipients and is hormonally induced (15). The ability of lymphocytes originating in the gut and sensitized to intestinal antigens to migrate to the mammary gland can account for the specificity of milk IgA against intestinal microorganisms and the consequent passive protection of the breast-fed infants. Ingestion of antigens during the third trimester of pregnancy can result in the appearance of colostral antibodies against these antigens—this process has been referred to as the enteromammary immune system (1), which forms part of the common mucosal system.

Within a few days after birth, the infant becomes colonized with indigenous bacteria. The early maternal-infant interactions are beneficial to the child not only in terms of emotional adjustment and the initiation of breast-feeding, but also in relation to optimal colonization of intestinal tract and skin. Colonization of the alimentary tract differs in infants fed on cow's milk or human milk. The bacterial population is predominantly *Lactobacillus bifidus* in the breast-fed, whereas the intestinal flora of babies fed on cow's milk is made mainly of gram-negative bacteria. The breast-fed infants are well protected, having acquired the mother's strains and getting breast milk rich in antibodies against those strains. Most outbreaks of epidemic diarrhea in maternity-unit nurseries appeared where neonates were separated from their mothers and bottle-fed. Breast-fed infants either did not contract the disease or, if they did, were able to conquer the infection, whereas, many formula-fed babies died.

Acute necrotizing enterocolitis described in 1974 appears to be related not only to prematurity, but to perinatal hypoxia and to lack of breast milk, even if the etiology seems to be an infection of the intestinal wall damaged by oxygen lack, by *Klebsiella*, or gram-negative organisms. This relatively common illness in other countries is, however, very rare in Czechoslovakia in spite of the low rate of breast-feeding.

INFLUENCE OF ARTIFICIAL ORAL COLONIZATION ON THE SYSTEMIC AND LOCAL ANTIBODY RESPONSE IN THE INTESTINE AND BREAST

In the clinical part of our work, the influence of artificial oral colonization with the nonenteropathogenic *E. coli* strain 083 on the systemic and local humoral antibody response in the intestine and the mammary gland was investigated. Maternal milk cells were isolated and their characteristics and functions studied in naturally colonized and artificially colonized infants.

The substitution of the randomly acquired intestinal flora by a tested nonenteropathogenic *E. coli* strain permits investigation of the immune reactions and keeps the composition of the intestinal flora partly under control (16).

The strain *E. coli* 083 was proved to be nonpathogenic in colostrum-deprived, germ-free, newborn piglets. It has favorable antigenic properties and, in our environment, does not occur as a spontaneous type. According to its biochemical properties, it is a normal classic *E. coli* strain, having no K antigen and not producing enterotoxin, as was confirmed by the WHO reference laboratory in Copenhagen. By using two different electrophoretic methods, it has been proven that the strain *E. coli* 083 does not carry any plasmid. The frequence of transfer of a transferable R plasmid, resistant to antibiotics, from an effective donor to *E. coli* 083 is 100 times lower if compared with that of a standard strain *E. coli* 600.

Twenty-five breast-fed and 25 formula-fed infants were colonized by oral administration of the strain *E. coli* 083. A living suspension was prepared from a 24-hr culture containing 5×10^8 organisms/ml. One milliliter was given to each child during the first 24 hr after birth and again 3 times a week for 4 successive weeks. Twenty breast-fed and 13 formula-fed infants were followed as controls. Samples of blood and feces were collected from the infants and mothers before colonization and at 2-week intervals after colonization up to 24 weeks of life. Milk samples were taken from the mothers every fortnight during the time of breast-feeding. Smears from the infant's mouth were checked bacteriologically 24 hr after each administration of the suspension. Specific antibodies against *E. coli* 083 in serum, stool filtrates, and milk samples were determined by passive hemagglutination, secretory IgA levels in stool filtrates and milk by radial immunodiffusion.

In another group of 11 mothers of colonized infants and 11 control mothers, milk cells in samples taken between the 8th and 23rd days after colonization were isolated according to the method described by Parmely et al. (22). The presence of cells producing or releasing antibodies was detected by the plaque technique. Both direct and indirect plaques were detected, the indirect ones after potentiation with anti-IgA and anti-IgA antibodies (30) using four different antigens coupled to sheep red blood cells (SRBC)-standard set *E. coli* 083, a mixture of *E. coli* types isolated from stools of mothers whose infants were colonized, from stools of control mothers, and from the stools of the colonized infants.

All infants were kept at the Department for Healthy Infants from birth until the age of six months. Informed consent was obtained from the parents.

The strain of *E. coli* 083 was detected in stool samples 48 hr after colonization of the infants and predominated over the other spontaneously acquired *E. coli* strains for several weeks (Fig. 3). The *E. coli* 083 was also found in all smears taken from the mouth of colonized infants and in some samples of the mother's milk. However, it was never detected in the mother's stool.

Colonization evoked a higher serum antibody response in both colonized groups of infants than in the control groups. The difference was significant from the 2nd to 8th week after colonization. Later, the titers of the two groups did not differ (Fig. 4).

In stool filtrates, higher titers of hemagglutinating copro-antibodies against *E. coli* 083 were detected in the colonized infants from the 2nd week after colonization. In breast-fed infants, however, the titers decreased after the 4th week, whereas in formula-fed infants the values remained high for 20 weeks if compared with the controls (Fig. 5).

Secretory IgA in stool filtrates measured by immunodiffusion was high in colonized breast-fed and formula-fed infants as well as in breast-fed controls, during the 2nd, 4th, 6th, and 8th week. Later, in breast-fed controls the levels

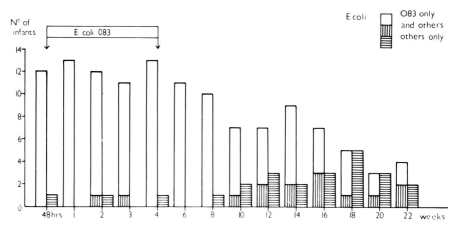

FIG. 3. Colonization of the intestine with *E. coli* 083 and other *E. coli* strains. Bacteriological findings.

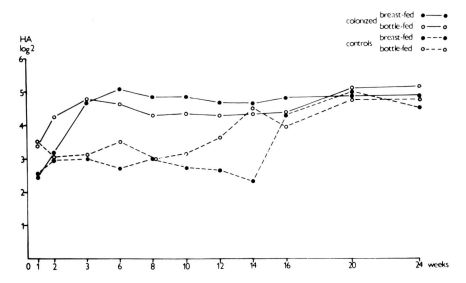

FIG. 4. Hemagglutinating antibody against *E. coli* 083 in the infant's serum. There are significant differences (*P* < 0.05) between the 6th and 12th week.

decreased to values found in formula-fed controls, while in both colonized groups the values still remained significantly high until 20 weeks (Fig. 6).

The level of hemagglutinating antibody against *E. coli* 083 in milk samples from mothers of the colonized infants was significantly higher during the 2nd,

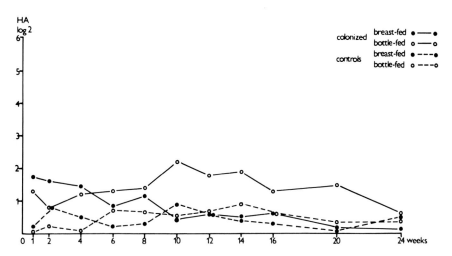

FIG. 5. Hemagglutinating antibody against *E. coli* 083 in stool filtrates. Significant differences (*P* < 0.01–0.05) are present at 2, 4, 10, 14, and 20 weeks after colonization.

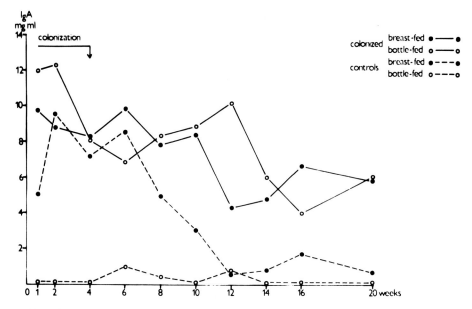

FIG. 6. Secretory IgA levels in stool filtrates. There are significant differences (*P* < 0.01–0.05) between the 2nd and 12th week after colonization.

4th, and 8th week after colonization than in milk of the control mothers. The values of total IgA in milk were not influenced by colonization (Fig. 7).

The cellular response demonstrated by the number of hemolytic plaques was higher in the mother's milk of colonized infants against both *E. coli* 083

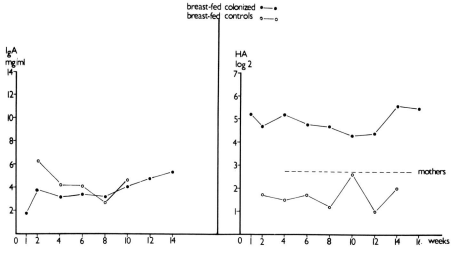

FIG. 7. Secretory IgA levels (*left*) and hemagglutinating antibodies against *E. coli* 083 (*right*) in the milk of mothers of colonized infants and control mothers. Hemagglutinating antibodies at 4, 6, and 8 weeks (*P* < 0.01).

antigens (i.e., the standard and the one isolated from the infant's stool), than in milk of control mothers, especially after potentiation with the IgA antiserum. No potentiation occurred when IgG antibody was used, nor did plaques develop against noncoated erythrocytes.

The cellular composition of the center of the plaques consisted of clusters of cells microscopically identified mainly as macrophages and noncellular particles coated with fat (Fig. 8). Figure 9 shows a comparison of the number of plaques in breast milk from colonized infants and controls.

The serum and local antibody response induced by oral colonization confirms the results of many authors who demonstrated antibody production after oral vaccination (26). In our study, as in germ-free piglets (28), a living strain was used for colonization which remained in the intestine for a long period of time and represented a permanent antigenic stimulus. The antibody production became detectable sooner than after natural colonization, which was particularly significant in formula-fed infants. In breast-fed infants, the response as far as IgA was concerned was masked by the massive supply from the maternal milk. Antibodies against Enterobacteriaceae do not cross the placenta and the newborn infant is, therefore, not protected against infections caused by those microbes, especially if deprived of breast-feeding. The early induction of antibodies in the intestine might provide local protection against gastrointestinal infections. We used the unusual ability of the strain *E. coli* 083 to persist in the intestine for a long time to demonstrate that it displaces already present pathogens and prevents their spreading into the gut (18).

The ability of the mammary gland to produce specific antibodies was proved by Goldblum et al. (8) in mothers colonized with the same *E. coli* strain 083 as we used in the infants. The precursors of the IgA-producing cells are thought not to be of local origin, but to have emigrated from the intestinal lymphatic tissue after having been sensitized by antigens present in the intestine. In our study, however, the infants were colonized and the absence of *E. coli* 083 in the mother's stool was repeatedly proved. Even in this model situation, the mammary gland displayed a specific antibody response. Recently, we also

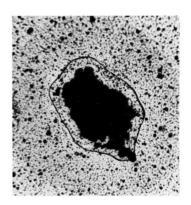

FIG. 8. Photomicrograph of a large lipid-laden macrophage in the center of a hemolytic plaque surrounded by fat particles. ×1200.

BREAST - MILK CELLS

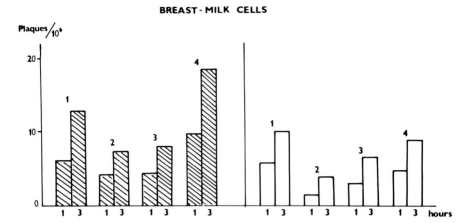

FIG. 9. Cellular response of the breast after antigenic stimulation with *E. coli*. **Left:** Colonized infants. **Right:** Controls. **Antigens:** 1, E. coli 083; 2, mixture of *E. coli* strains from mothers of colonized infants; 3, mixture of *E. coli* strains from control mothers; 4, *E. coli* from colonized infants.

found a higher antibody titer against *E. coli* 083 in the serum of the mothers of colonized infants than against their own *E. coli* isolated from stool samples. We assume, therefore, that the antibody response of the mammary gland is induced by penetration of the antigen, repeatedly found in the infant's mouth as well as in the milk of the mothers, into the breast macrophages presenting the antigen to lymphocytes. The possible role of subepithelially localized lymphocytes present in the mammary gland and/or migrating cells in the process of specific antibody formation against locally administered antigen cannot be excluded. Campbell et al. (4) have also shown that *Salmonella* organisms introduced into the mouth of the suckling calf lead to raised antibodies against these bacteria in the cow's milk. They suggested a mechanism of diathelic immunization of the mammary gland which is capable of producing specific antibodies in response to pathogens reaching the breast tissue from the lacteal duct. The antibodies are protecting the gastrointestinal tract and such mechanism can be specific for each mother-infant pair (4).

Ahlstedt et al. demonstrated milk cells actively producing IgA antibodies by indirect plaque formation using anti-IgA and antisecretory component sera (1). However, they did not use morphologic methods confirming the type of the central cell in the plaque. Also, the ratio of 8% of plaque-forming cells to the total amount of cells seems to be high—it would mean that nearly all lymphoid cells are producers of plaques. In the work of Crago et al. (6) dealing with the character of colostral cells, macrophages are described as the main cells containing IgA. Pittard et al. (24) demonstrated macrophages that pinocytose immunoglobulins from the milk and release them gradually.

We may also suggest from our results that the elements present in the center of the hemolytic plaques and analyzed microscopically are macrophages, noncellular globules, and polymorphonuclear leukocytes coated with fat. They are forming more hemolytic plaques against erythrocytes coated with *E. coli* 083 antigen than against *E. coli* antigens prepared from the mother's stool. Mestecky et al. (20) demonstrated hemolytic plaques formed by macrophages and noncellular milk globules against different *E. coli* antigens. Immunoglobulins detected in those elements are thought to originate in the environment. The origin and mode of acquisition of immunoglobulins by these globular elements and phagocytic cells remain unclear.

The fact that milk fat plays a role in the immunologic mechanisms of the milk was demonstrated by Wiman et al. (32). They detected histocompatible antigens in the membranes of the milk fat globules. In our hemolytic plaques, we could always demonstrate the presence of fat around the cellular or noncellular elements present in the center of the plaques.

The possibility of stimulating the mammary gland to increase the antibody production has a direct practical importance since the breast-fed infant swallows the antibodies and cells and they afford the infant a better local protection. Thus, it is not only the breast milk that is important, but it is the process of breast-feeding that provides the immunologic protection and the antigenic stimulation followed by local immune response of the breast as another possible mechanism of protection.

REFERENCES

1. Ahlstedt, S., Carlsson, B., Hanson, L. A., and Goldblum, R. M. (1975): Antibody production by human colostral cells. *Scand. J. Immunol.*, 4:535–539.
2. Boackle, R. J., Pruitt, K. M., and Mestecky, J. (1974): The interaction of human complement with artificially aggregated preparation of human secretory IgA. *Immunochemistry*, 11:543–548.
3. Bullen, J. J. (1976): Iron-binding proteins and other factors in milk responsible for resistance to *E. coli. Ciba Foundation Symposium No. 42*, p. 149. Elsevier, Amsterdam.
4. Campbell, B., Sarvaw, M., and Peterson, W. E. (1957): Diathelic immunization: a maternal offspring relationship involving milk antibodies. *Science (NY)*, 125:932–937.
5. Chandra, R. K. (1978): Immunological aspects of human milk. *Nutr. Rev.*, 36:265–272.
6. Crago, S. S., Prince, S. J., Pretlow, T. G., McGhee, J. R., and Mestecky, J. (1979): Human colostral cells. I. Separation and characterization. *Clin. Exp. Immunol.*, 38:585–597.
7. Fomon, S. J. (1974): *Infant Nutrition*, 2nd ed. Saunders, Philadelphia.
8. Goldblum, R. M., Ahlstedt, S., Carlsson, B., Hanson, L. A., Jodal, U., Lidin-Janson, G., and Sahl, A. (1975): Antibody forming cells in human colostrum after oral immunization. *Nature*, 257:797–799.
9. Gyorgy, P. S. (1971): Biochemical aspects of human milk. *Am. J. Clin. Nutr.*, 24:976.
10. Haed, J. R., and Beer, A. E. (1979): *In vivo* and *in vitro* assessment of the immunologic role of leukocytic cells in milk. In: *Immunology of Breast Milk*, edited by P. L. Ogra and D. Dayton, p. 207. Raven Press, New York.
11. Halsey, J. F., Johnson, B. H., and Cebra, J. J. (1980): Transport of immunoglobulins from serum into colostrum. *J. Exp. Med.*, 151:767–772.
12. Hambraeus, L., Forsum, E., and Lonnerdal, B. (1975): Nutritional aspects of breast milk and cow's milk formulas. In: *Food and Immunology*, edited by L. Hambraeus, L. Hanson, and H. MacFarlane, p. 116. Almquist and Wiksell, Stockholm.
13. Hanson, L. A., Carlsson, B., Gruz, J. R., Gracia, B., Holmgren, J., Khan, S. R., Lindbland, B. S., Svennerholm, A. M., Svennerholm, B., and Urrutia, J. (1979): Immune response in the mammary gland. In: *Immunology of Breast Milk*, edited by P. L. Ogra and D. Dayton, p. 145. Raven Press, New York.
14. Jellife, D. B. (1978): *Human Milk in the Modern World*, edited by D. B. Jellife and P. Jellife. University Press, Oxford.

15. Lamm, M. D., Weisz-Carrington, P., Roux, M. E., McWilliams, M., and Philips-Quagliata, J. M. (1978): Development of the IgA system in the mammary gland. In: *Secretory Immunity and Infection*, edited by J. McGhee, J. Mestecky, and J. L. Babb, p. 35. Plenum Press, New York.

16. Lodinova, R., Jouja, V., and Wagner, V. (1973): Serum immunoglobulins and copro-antibody formation in infants after artificial intestinal colonization with *Escherichia coli* 083 and oral lysozyme administration. *Pediatr. Res.*, 7:659–669.

17. Lodinova, R., and Jouja, V. (1977): Antibody production by the mammary gland in mothers after artificial oral colonization of their infants with a nonpathogenic strain *E. coli* 083. *Acta Paediatr. Scand.*, 66:705–708.

18. Lodinova, R., Jouja, V., Vinšova, N., and Vocel, J. (1980): New attempts and possibilities in prevention and treatment of intestinal coli-infections in infants. *Czech. Med.*, 3:47–58.

19. Mestecky, J., McGhee, J. R., Crago, S. S., Jackson, S., Kilian, M., Kiyono, H., Babb, J. L., and Michalek, S. M. (1980): Molecular-cellular interactions in the secretory IgA response. *J. Reticuloendoth. Soc.*, (Suppl.), 28:45s–60s.

20. Mestecky, J., Crago, S. S., Laven, G. T., and McGhee, J. R. (1981): Immunoglobulin containing cells and noncellular elements in human colostrum. In: *The Mucosal Immune System in Health and Disease*, edited by P. L. Ogra and J. Bienenstock. *Proceedings of the Eighty-First Ross Conference on Pediatric Research.* Columbus, Ohio.

21. Ogra, S. S., Weintraub, D. I., and Ogra, P. L. (1978): Immunologic aspects of human colostrum and milk: Interaction with the intestinal immunity of the neonate. In: *Secretory Immunity and Infection*, edited by J. McGhee, J. Mestecky, and J. L. Babb, p. 95. Plenum Press, New York-London.

22. Parmely, M. J., Beer, A. E., and Billingham, R. E. (1976): *In vitro* studies on the T-lymphocyte population of human milk. *J. Exp. Med.*, 144:358–370.

23. Parmely, M. J., and Beer, A. E. (1977): Colostral cell mediated immunity and the concept of a common secretory immune system. *J. Dairy Sci.*, 60:655–665.

24. Pittard, W. B., Polmar, S. H., and Fanroff, A. A. (1977): The breast milk macrophage: A potential vehicle for immunoglobulin transport. *J. Reticuloendoth. Soc.*, 22:597–603.

25. Porter, P. (1979): Adoptive immunization of the neonate by breast factors. In: *Immunology of Breast Milk*, edited by P. L. Ogra and D. Dayton, p. 197. Raven Press, New York.

26. Raettig, H. (1978): Orale Immunisierung mit nichtvermehrungsfahigen Mikroorganismen oder ihren Antigenen. 19. Mitteilung: Feldversuche mit polyvalenten Enteritis-Oral-Impfstoffen. *Abl. Bakt. Hyg.*, I abt. Orig. A 242:31–41.

27. Sterzl, J., and Riha, I. (1965): Detection of cells producing 7S antibodies by the plaque technique. *Nature*, 208:858–859.

28. Tlaskalova, H., Sterzl, J., Hajek, P., Pospisil, M., Riha, I., Marvanova, H., Kamarytova, V., Mandel, L., Kruml, J., and Kovaru, F. (1970): The development of antibody formation during embryonal and postnatal periods. In: *Developmental Aspects of Antibody Formation and Structure*, edited by J. Sterzl and I. Riha, p. 767. Academia, Prague.

29. Tlaskalova, H., Rejnek, J., Travnicek, J., and Lanc, A. (1970): The effect of antibodies present in the intestinal tract of germfree piglets on the infection caused by intravenous administration of the pathogenic strain *Escherichia coli* 055. *Folia Microb.*, 15:372–376.

30. Tlaskalova-Hogenova, H., Cerna, J., and Mandel, L. (1981): Peroral immunization of germfree piglets: Appearance of antibody-forming cells and antibodies of different isotypes. *Scand. J. Immunol.*, 13:467–472.

31. Walker, A. W. (1979): Antigen penetration across the immature gut: Effect of immunologic and maturation factors in colostrum. In: *Immunology of Breast Milk*, edited by P. L. Ogra and D. Dayton, pp. 227–234. Raven Press, New York.

32. Wiman, K., Curman, B., and Peterson, P. A. (1979): Demonstration of HLA-DR-like antigens on milk fat globule membranes. *Eur. J. Immunol.*, 9:190–195.

33. Great Britain Department of Health and Social Security (1977): *The Composition of Mature Human Milk*, Report of a Working Party of the Committee on Medical Aspects of Food Policy—Report on Health and Social Subjects, No. 12. HMSO, London.

Acute Diarrhea: Its Nutritional Consequences in Children, edited by J. A. Bellanti.
Nestlé, Vevey/Raven Press, New York © 1983.

ROLE OF BREAST-FEEDING IN THE NUTRITIONAL STATUS OF INFANTS

Comments

Benjamin José Schmidt

Department of Puericulture and Social Pediatrics, Escola Paulista de Medicina, Federal University, São Paulo, Brazil

This chapter reports chiefly on our epidemiological studies that have been conducted over the last 14 years in the lowest socioeconomic classes of our Latin American communities.

The specific concerns of this chapter are the epidemiological studies of breast-feeding that are being conducted in several areas of eight Latin American countries[1] and in Portugal since 1981 under the coordination of the Latin American Pediatrics Association (ALAPE). All data will be available soon; those regarding the six Brazilian state capitals (Natal, Salvador, Sao Paulo, Belo Horizonte, Rio de Janeiro, Florianopolis) have already been computer-analyzed. As far as the role of breast-feeding in acute diarrhea is concerned, I would like to comment on the correlations between the length of breast-feeding, the ingestion of colostrum, as well as the time elapsed between birth and the beginning of breast-feeding and the incidence of acute diarrhea and/or dehydration within one or more of the following periods: early neonatal (0–7 days), late neonatal (8–30 days), 1 to 6 months, and 7 to 12 months.

Of a total number of 2,545 children, data on the length of breast-feeding could be collected on 2,386 cases. Of these, 220 children had never been breast-fed, 446 received breast milk for less than a month, 298 until the end of the first month, 369 until the end of the 2nd month, 348 until the end of the 3rd month, and 173, 113, and 125, respectively, until the end of the 4th, 5th, and 6th months of life. Up to the period comprised between the 7th and 12th month of life, 291 were breast-fed.

Children who took colostrum numbered 2,151 (88.0%), while 175 (12.0%) did not take it. As for the beginning of breast-feeding, of 2,297 children, 298 were first fed within the first 6 hr after birth, 601 between 7 and 12 hr, 871 between 13 and 24 hr, 266 between 25 and 48 hr, 193 between the end of the 2nd and the 4th day of life, 36 between the 5th and 7th day, and 32 on the 8th day or later.

---

[1] Coordinators of the studied areas: H. Bezerra (Natal), N.C.A. Barros (Salvador), B. J. Schmidt (S. Paulo), C. M. Menezes (Belo Horizonte), R. M. Martins (Rio de Janeiro), and N. Grisard (Florianópolis).

The correlations between these various parameters and the incidence of diarrhea and/or dehydration were as follows:

1. During the early neonatal period: The incidence of children with diarrhea was 40 out of the 2,386 children studied. Of the 666 children who were never breast-fed or were breast-fed during the first days of life only, 18 (2.70%) had diarrhea. On the other hand, of the 1,720 children who were breast-fed, 22 (1.28%) had diarrhea. As for dehydration, 11 out of the 2,386 children studied presented it, 5 (0.75%) of these 11 children belonged to the group who were never breast-fed or breast-fed only during the first days of life; the other 6 (0.34%) belonged to the group of children which received breast milk.

2. During the late neonatal period: Of the total number of 2,243 children, 81 had diarrhea and 25 had dehydration. Of the 81 with diarrhea, 37 (6.25%) out of 592 children had never received breast milk or had received it for less than the first 30 days of life. The remaining 44 represent 2.66% of the 1,651 children who were breast-fed.

Of the 25 children with dehydration, 11 (1.85%) belonged to the group of 592 children who were never breast-fed or were breast-fed for less than the first 30 days, while 14 (0.84%) belonged to the group of breast-fed children.

3. Period from 1 to 6 months: Of a total number of 2,063 children, 294 had diarrhea; of these, 258 (14.4%) belonged to the group of 1,780 children who had received breast milk from the first till the end of the 6th month of life, while 36 (12.7%) belonged to the group of 283 children who were breast-fed up to the 7th month or longer.

4. Period of 7 to 12 months: Of a total number of 1,061 children, 119 had diarrhea; 91 of these belonged to the group of 814 children (11.1%) who had been breast-fed for less than 7 months, while the other 28 children belonged to the group of 247 children (11.3%) who received breast milk up to the period of between the 7th and the 12th month of life.

Forty children of the 1,061 had dehydration; 32 of them belonged to the group of 814 children (3.9%) who had been breast-fed for less than 7 months, while the other 8 belonged to the group of 247 children (3.2%) who received breast milk up to the period of between the 7th and 12th months of life.

The correlations between the ingestion of colostrum and the incidence of diarrhea and/or dehydration were as follows:

In the early and late neonatal periods, there was a clear-cut decrease of the diarrhea and/or dehydration incidence in the children who took colostrum, as compared to those who did not. Yet in the period from 1 to 6 months and from 7 to 12 months, the influence of colostrum ingestion on the incidence of diarrhea and/or dehydration was not important.

Regarding the time elapsed between birth and the beginning of breast-feeding and its correlation with the incidence of diarrhea and/or dehydration, the data obtained from our sample were variable, not allowing firm conclusions.

The results obtained, so far, from our study confirm the importance of breast milk for reducing the incidence of diarrhea and dehydration, particularly during the first 30 days of life, even in children coming from the lowest socio-economic levels of developing countries such as Brazil.

Acute Diarrhea: Its Nutritional Consequences in Children, edited by J. A. Bellanti.
Nestlé, Vevey/Raven Press, New York © 1983.

ROLE OF BREAST-FEEDING IN THE NUTRITIONAL STATUS OF INFANTS

Discussion

Dr. Pierce: I think there is now a rather large body of evidence, from a variety of animal species and also from humans, to indicate that parental immunization, even in the instance of prior enteric priming is clearly a two-edged sword.

There are a number of studies that show what Dr. Hanson reports, namely, one can prime enterically and boost an IgA response by parental antigens.

I think it is important to carry those observations further, because there is evidence that parental immunization also stimulates very potent suppressor mechanisms which, with time, tend to become the dominant effect of parental immunization so that two effects are seen. First, the duration of the IgA response at mucosal level, which is stimulated by parental antigen, is brief compared with an IgA response stimulated by local boosting. Second, if one attempts to repeat that effect by parental immunization again after some weeks or some months, one gets either no response or a much reduced response.

Dr. Koster and I have shown in rats, for example, that the mechanisms involved in parental suppression of mucosal and immune responses are complex; they certainly involve suppressor lymphocyte mediation and they may, under certain circumstances, also involve a suppression by serum IgG antibodies.

It is important to recognize that the anatomy and the design of the mucosal system appear clearly designed to respond to mucosal-applied antigens. Also, just as mucosal application of antigens may stimulate tolerance to subsequent parental immunization, there is now growing evidence that parental immunization may stimulate tolerance to mucosal entities.

Dr. Hanson: I would like to ask Dr. Mata if in the studies he has done in his country and elsewhere he has seen better protection with breast milk than Dr. Schmidt's data suggest, given the same cultural need to administer water, apple juice, and whatever else might be needed for the baby early in life.

Dr. Mata: I think everyone here was impressed with Dr. Schmidt's data showing not the kind of protection we would like to see with breast-feeding, relative to the occurrence of diarrhea. The question is whether this is due to the introduction into the diet of large quantities of pathogens by nonformula food. In practically all cultures, even if the infant has been well breast-fed, they are always given small amounts of other things. It is natural to give things like honey. Many of these products are contaminated.

In one of our studies, we recorded data on the incidence of diarrhea in specifically breast-fed babies and in those who had received supplemental food. The diarrhea rate in the first 6 months of the year was measured by nurses or in the homes. There was eight times the incidence of diarrhea in the weaned children as opposed to those who were specifically breast-fed, and in those who were breast-fed and received supplemental meals. There is no doubt there is a protection from breast milk, itself, alone.

Dr. Levine: We have generated some data recently in humans that are of some importance concerning the question of parental vaccine and stimulation of local antibody.

Usually, we work with vaccines that are given by the oral route. But, in this instance, we happened to be working with parenteral vaccines in United States young adults. The vaccine consisted of purified type 1 pelli from an *E. coli* strain. We collected intestinal fluid before immunization from these 9 young adults. They were given two doses of parenteral vaccine, 1 month apart. We collected intestinal fluid again 1 week after the second dose, and then 3 weeks thereafter. We found that nobody had antibody in his or her intestinal fluid prior to immunization with this vaccine, and a week after the second dose, there was a striking response in 8 of 9 individuals. There was also a serum antibody response, the kinetics of which suggested that everybody was primed to type 1 somatic pelli. Therefore, this is one example that would corroborate the findings in Pakistani women by Lars Hanson and his co-workers, with respect to parenteral vaccine giving very striking local antibody responses in primed individuals.

By no means do we push the use of this parenteral vaccine, but it is a phenomenon that is corroborated, and it is worth mentioning.

THERAPY AND PREVENTION

*Acute Diarrhea: Its Nutritional Consequences
in Children*, edited by J. A. Bellanti.
Nestlé, Vevey/Raven Press, New York © 1983.

NUTRITIONAL BENEFITS RELATED TO ORAL THERAPY

An Overview

David R. Nalin

*International Health Program and Department of Epidemiology and Preventive
Medicine, University of Maryland College of Medicine, Baltimore, Maryland 21201*

The subject of oral therapy's nutritional effects is still somewhat controversial due to apparent inconsistencies between findings of different investigators and even of the same investigators in different studies. Moreover, the complex and costly nature of longitudinal studies of nutritional impact has permitted completion of relatively few such studies to date. While the data do not yet permit definitive conclusions, it is useful to analyze aspects of conceptualization, design, and methodology that may explain the variations in results, to review briefly the available studies, and to examine some directions that future studies might usefully take.

It is important to define exactly what is meant by "oral therapy." Oral therapy in the current context can be defined as a treatment modality which provides a rational, physiologically based, and effective means of replacing by mouth the losses—of water, electrolytes, and nutrients—accruing due to attacks of acute, watery diarrhea. This broad definition encompasses the main functions of oral therapy, including the deficit replacement and the maintenance phases of water and electrolyte replacement, and the maintenance and repair phases of nutritional rehabilitation of the patient with acute, watery diarrhea. The concept of oral therapy defined in this manner considers both water and electrolyte balance and nutritional balance throughout the course of acute diarrhea and during the convalescent and postconvalescent phases. In applying this concept, different investigators have used different approaches, comparison of which is facilitated by segregating the different components of oral therapy including different formulas, regimens, and methods used during the acute, convalescent, and postconvalescent phases, for both rehydration and maintenance of fluid and electrolyte balance and nutritional rehabilitation.

Before discussing the theoretical and the proven nutritional benefits of oral therapy, it is useful to briefly review the nutritional effects of acute, watery diarrhea (Table 1). Based on these effects, the expected theoretical benefits of oral therapy can be derived, as depicted in Table 2.

These classifications of oral therapy components and of relevant nutritional factors facilitate the development of a series of different aspects deserving

TABLE 1. *Nutritional effects of acute watery diarrhea*[a]

Nutritional effects	Mechanisms of effects
Reduced net oral intake	Anorexia Nausea Vomiting "Therapeutic" starvation
Gut response to acute watery diarrhea and to nutritional damage	
Maldigestion	↓Gut enzyme activity; ↓cell turnover pH Alterations Hypochlorhydria ↓ or ↑ Motility Indigestible products of bacterial breakdown of nutrients
Reduced absorptive capacity	↓Transit time Stasis (ileus) ?Direct bacterial and parasitic damage or toxin-mediated effects Mucosal damage Villous atrophy Chronic enteritis Effects of wrong therapies (neomycin)
Nutrient losses into gut	Protein-losing enteropathies GI bleeding
Competition for nutrients	Gut parasitic and bacterial overgrowth Chronic persistent colonization
Increased catabolism	Fever Stress Hormonal responses
Increased caloric utilization	↑Energy expenditure ↑Requirements for repair
Decreased feeding efficiency	↓Muscle strength due to potassium loss (↓sucking strength, ↓breast manipulation, ↑sibling competition for food)
Skeletal deformities	Potassium deprivation

investigation in relation to oral therapy's nutritional benefits (Table 3). The nutritional impact of these variables would occur during the acute, convalescent, or postconvalescent phases (Table 4). Fortunately, these complexities can be reduced to two major possibilities (Table 5), of which the first seems self-evident; one would expect that variations in outcome between different studies of related or dependent variables would depend chiefly on details of study design, patient selection, and execution. The second of these possibilities, i.e., that differences in the extent of nutritional benefits found by different workers are attributable to specific variations in formula composition, is intriguing; I would propose that of these variables, the one most likely to promote significant long-term nutritional benefit is prevention of significant potassium deficits

TABLE 2. *Theoretical expected nutritional benefits of oral therapy*

Expected benefit	Mechanisms of benefit
Restore net oral intake toward normal	Encourage uninterrupted oral intake Discourage "starvation therapy" Reduce vomiting and anorexia
Ameliorate maldigestion and reconstitute gastric-acid barrier	Avoid ↓ enzyme activity Promote enzyme induction by early feeding Promote normal gastric acid secretion by avoiding nutritional deficiencies; ↑ gut cell turnover ?"Flushing out" effect of bacteria, parasites, or their toxins
Raise absorptive capacity	Normalize gut motility ↓Risk of ileus & stasis and bacterial overgrowth by K^+ replacement (Antibiotics and antiparasitics)
Decrease competition for nutrients	(Antibiotics and antiparasitics)
Decrease catabolism	↓Fever; ↓stress ↑Hormonal status ↑Protein synthesis
Decrease caloric expenditure	↑Rest and relaxation ↓Muscular exertion (crying, expressing thirst or hunger by movement)
↑Feeding efficacy	Volume replacement K^+ replacement ↑Muscle strength for feeding
Improve maternal-child relationships and interaction	Avoid "sickly baby" syndrome Encourage feeding by mother
Educate on food and personal hygiene Avoid inappropriate therapies which cause malabsorption and anorexia	↓Gut exposure to pathogens, i.e., ↓neomycin use

during and after acute, watery diarrhea episodes through the use of oral solution formulas relatively rich in potassium. Such formulas should, by correcting and avoiding potassium deficits, help improve strength for feeding, including breast manipulation and sucking strength of infants; this improved strength should help improve maternal-child interactions, both physical and psychological.

In addition, the Philippine data of Dr. Hirschhorn and colleagues (10,11) showing a significantly lower nutritional benefit in terms of weight gain after oral rehydration therapy using a sucrose-electrolyte oral solution formula compared to that achieved using a glucose-electrolyte formula bear repetition. These data suggest that the nutritional benefits seen with oral glucose-electrolyte formulas might not be seen after oral salt-sugar (so-called "incomplete" formulas). This would be consistent with the earlier work of Torres-Pinedos and colleagues (20).

The studies of oral therapy's nutritional benefits to date have focused on the relative benefits of rapid refeeding versus starvation therapy of diarrhea

TABLE 3. *Various aspects of oral therapy's nutritional benefits to be investigated*

Therapy	Nutritionally relevant variables
ORS[a] formula	$\uparrow K^+$ vs $\downarrow K^+$ Glucose alone vs glucose + glycine (13,14,17) Sucrose vs glucose Addition of other substrates
ORS regimen	Postrehydration feeding vs prerehydration feeds 2:1 vs "straight" Postdiarrheal K^+ supplementation vs none Potassium chloride supplements vs dietary K^+ repair
ORS method	Type of instruction Packet vs spoon vs pinch, other ingredient measures Packet + instruction alone vs demonstration + packet + instruction Mother-participation in hospital and clinic therapy Supervision: depot-holder vs paramedical vs nurse vs doctor

Nutritional "formula"	Breast vs bottle (immune system or gut hormone benefits)
	One-half strength vs full-strength formulas
	Different formula compositions
	   High energy formulas
	   Vitamin and mineral supplements
	   Trace elements
	2:1 vs "straight" ORS::% dilution of milk feeds::Na^+ balance

Nutritional regimen	Alternate ORS/formula or breast (maintenance) Advancement rate (dilute → high energy feeds)
Nutritional method	Instruction modality Supplement modality (K^+-rich foods, postdiarrheal menu choice) Follow-up modality Feed frequency and amount
	Program management systems

[a] ORS = oral rehydration solution.

TABLE 4. *Mechanism of nutritional impact of oral rehydration*
therapy (ORT) by phase of illness

Illness phase	Mechanism
Acute	Restoration of circulatory volume, strength, rapid resumption of feeding
Convalescent	Avoid starvation, give nutritional maintenance Advance as tolerated to breast milk or to full or high-energy formulas Potassium replacement

Postconvalescent	Therapeutic interventions
	   Potassium supplementation
	   Vitamin and mineral repletion
	Nutritional instruction and motivation
	   $\uparrow$Hygiene in food handling and waste disposal
	   $\downarrow$Cumulative effects of multiple episodes
	   Avoidance of nutritional hypochlorhydria

patients, and on relative weight gain, both short- and long-term, when a given type of oral therapy is used instead of traditional or other therapies.

Present data (Table 6) indicate that (a) patients with diarrhea should be fed,

TABLE 5. *Oral therapy nutritional benefits*

Area	Nutritional benefits
Behavioral	Baby eats more, sooner and better, due to instructions, motivation, and encouragement of mother and health care workers
Physiologic	ORS formula itself enhances feeding and nutritional repair by physiologic mechanisms, i.e., K^+ replacement $\rightarrow$ ↑ strength or glycine + glucose $\rightarrow$ ↑ rate of cell repair, ↑ protein synthesis and ↑ gut cell turnover

not starved; (b) feeding should not be delayed, i.e., should start immediately after rehydration is complete, interrupted only intermittently during subsequent phases of additional maintenance water and electrolyte therapy by mouth; and (c) early feeding in the context of oral rehydration therapy using a glucose-electrolyte solution formula yields a greater short- and long-term weight gain than traditional therapies or nutritional advice alone. In studies conducted so far, however, the formulas used are not always clearly defined and the regimens used are often vaguely described; in general, methodology has been crude, albeit practical, based chiefly on serial weights and monitoring of changes in weight, supervised by technical and field staff, but with the precise content and quality of staff-mother interactions not reported.

We need to know the independent value of different formulas, regimens, and methods to determine how they compare or how they influence mechanisms governing nutritional outcome. This will enable us to identify the dominant variables promoting nutritional benefit and, by emphasizing them in diarrheal-disease control programs, to ensure consistency of optimal results in nutritional management of patients with acute, watery diarrhea. The addition of glycine or certain other amino acids to glucose in ORS should also promote long-term nutritional benefit by reducing the duration and volume of diarrhea (14,15). A study is needed to show whether this is due to increased absorption alone or to an enhancement of protein synthesis resulting in increased gut cell turnover which could hasten shedding of enterotoxin-affected gut mucosal epithelial cells.

TABLE 6. *Studies to date*

Question studied	Studies
Group I	
Starve or feed?	Feed[a]
Slow feed vs rapid feed	Feed early[b]
Group II	
Better weight gain after ORT?	Yes and no[c]
	Yes[d]
	No[e]

[a] Refs. 3, 12.
[b] Refs. 2, 4, 18, 19.
[c] Refs. 9, 10, 11.
[d] Refs. 1, 5, 6, 15; M. Coruh et al., *unpublished data*; L. El Sayyed et al., *unpublished data*.
[e] Ref. 16; A. Swamy et al., *unpublished data*.

It should be noted, however, that a number of these variables have been inadequately quantitated in the available studies based chiefly on field-worker's reports of mothers' impressions or recollections—notoriously unreliable data. This problem exists, for example, with regard to certain commonly used terms, such as "appetite" and "anorexia," and I would suggest that quantitative approaches should replace impressions as modes of measuring infant feeding patterns, and that terms too vague to permit replication of methods should be avoided. For example, frequency of acceptance and ingestion of foods offered at regular intervals, and amount consumed per unit time, would appear to be more satisfactory indicators of anorexia or appetite than a mother's recollections of her infant's variations in intake alone. One also wonders whose pleasure we mean by the often used term "ad libitum," Latin for "at pleasure," as applied to oral solution feeding regimens and methods. Do we mean the infant's pleasure, the mother's, the nurse's, or the doctor's? Is the infant given oral solution at every cry, when it moves around, when the mother feels like it, or when the nurse is back between coffee breaks? It takes two to rehydrate, and it would be helpful to describe, as precisely as possible, the actual methods used in the wards, clinics, and homes. Table 7 suggests some potentially useful indicators for measurement of these variables in a more quantitative way, which might help to identify the mechanisms of oral therapy's nutritional effects.

It can readily be appreciated that very few of the possible mechanisms by which oral therapy may benefit nutrition have been monitored or subjected to controlled clinical examination, and since the number of such mechanisms is large, this may account for variations in findings even from year to year, or study to study. Since a number of the relevant variables are of a subjective nature, their quantification demands a methodology appropriate to the study goals. Based on the studies completed to date, however, the following conclusions can be drawn:

TABLE 7. Potentially useful indicators of nutritional effects of diarrhea

Variable	Indicator
Anorexia	% and rate offered feeds are ingested
Nausea	Subjective reporting (interval questionning)
Vomiting	Direct bedside monitoring
↓Forced starvation	Weight and caloric density of foods taken
Gut enzymes	Biopsy, biochemical analysis
Gut pH	Intubation, aspiration pH measurement
Motility	Transit times
	Serial midabdominal girth (ileus)
Hypochlorhydria	Stomach acid production rates
Rinseout effect	Duration of diarrhea (e.g., ST enterotoxin)
↓Stress (energy expenditure)	Timed behavioral observations
	(% time crying or flailing arms vs calm)
Hormones	Plasma levels
Muscle strength	Suck strength; breast manipulation,
	frequency; transducer measurements
Maternal-child interaction	Graves' scores (7)
Education	Recall evaluation
Formula composition, concentration	Weight change

1. In most studies, oral therapy with early refeeding leads to increased weight gain, both short- and long-term.

2. The relative causal importance of motivational and behavioral changes versus physiologic effects resulting from oral therapy remains undefined.

3. Further studies to define the causal variables are needed in view of some unexplained negative findings and the importance of identifying and facilitating reproducibility of oral therapy's significant nutritional benefit.

BIBLIOGRAPHY

1. Barzgar, M. A., Ourshano, S., and Amini, J. N. (1980): The evaluation of the effectiveness of oral rehydration in acute diarrhea of children under three years of age in West Azerbaijan, Iran. *J. Trop. Pediatr.*, 26:217–222.
2. Chung, A. W. (1948): The effect of oral feeding at different levels on the absorption of foodstuffs in infantile diarrhea. *J. Pediatr.*, 33(1):1–13.
3. Chung, A. W., and Viscorova, B. (1948): The effect of early oral feeding versus early oral starvation on the course of infantile diarrhea. *J. Pediatr.*, 32:14–22.
4. Dugdale, A., Lovell, S., Gibbs, V., and Ball, D. (1982): Refeeding after acute gastroenteritis: a controlled study. *Arch. Dis. Child.*, 57:76–78.
5. Egemen, A., and Bertan, M. (1980): A study of oral rehydration therapy by midwives in a rural area near Ankara. *Bull. WHO*, 58:333–338.
6. El Sherbini, A. F., Fahmy, S. I., Eid, E. E., Goda, M. Y., El Tantawy, A. S., and El Sayyed, L. (1978): The use of oral rehydration in infantile diarrhea. *J. Egypt. Public Health Assoc.*, 53 (Suppl. 5–6):82–104.
7. Graves, P. L. (1976): Nutrition, infant behavior and maternal characteristics: A pilot study in West Bengal, India. *Am. J. Clin. Nutr.*, 29: 305–319.
8. Hirschhorn, N., and Denny, K. M. (1975): Oral glucose-electrolyte therapy for diarrhea: a means to maintain or improve nutrition? *Am. J. Clin. Nutr.*, 28:189–192.
9. International Study Group (1977): A positive effect on the nutrition of Philippine children of an oral glucose-electrolyte solution given at home for the treatment of diarrhea. *Bull. WHO*, 55:87–94.
10. International Study Group (1981): Beneficial effects of oral electrolyte-sugar solutions in the treatment of children's diarrhea. *J. Trop. Pediatr.*, 27:62–68.
11. International Study Group (1981): Beneficial effects of oral electrolyte-sugar solutions in the treatment of children's diarrhoea. 2. Studies in seven villages. *J. Trop. Pediatr.*, 27:136–140.
12. Molla, A., Molla, A. M., Rahim, A., Sarker, S. A., Mozaffar, Z., and Rahaman, M. (1980): Intake and absorption of nutrients in children with cholera and rotavirus infection during acute diarrhea and after recovery. *ICDDR, B.*, Dacca.
13. Nalin, D. R., and Cash, R. A. (1970): Oral or nasogastric maintenance therapy for diarrheas of unknown etiology resembling cholera. *Trans. R. Soc. Trop. Med. Hyg.*, 64:769–771.
14. Nalin, D. R., Cash, R. A., Rahaman, M., and Yunus, M. (1970): Effect of glycine and glucose on sodium and water absorption in patients with cholera. *Gut*, 11:768–772.
15. Pal, S. C. (1978): In: *Annual Report, National Institute of Cholera and Enteric Diseases*, pp. 3–4. Calcutta.
16. Rowland, M. G. M., and Cole, T. J. (1980): The effect of early glucose-electrolyte therapy on diarrhea and growth in rural Gambian village children. *J. Trop. Pediatr.*, 26:54, 57.
17. Sim, A. J. W., Wolfe, B. M., Young, V. R., Clarke, D., and Moore, F. D. (1979): Glucose promotes whole-body protein synthesis from infused aminoacids in fasting man. *Lancet*, i:68–72.
18. Soenarto, A. H., Suprapto, Sutrisno, D. S., Sebodo, T., Radjiman and Lahmuddin (1979): Milk lactose: the amount tolerated in post diarrheal children *Trop. Pediatr. Environ. Child Health*, 104–106 (Aug.)
19. Soeprapto, Yati-Soenarto, Nelwan, Moenginah, P. A. and Ismangoen, (1979): Feeding children with diarrhea. *Trop. Pediatr. Environ. Child Health*, 25:97–100.
20. Torres-Pinedo, R., Lavastida, M., Rivera, C. L., Rodriguez, H., and Ortiz, A. (1966): Studies on infant diarrhea. I. A comparison of the effects of milk feeding and intravenous therapy upon the composition and volume of the stool and urine. *J. Clin. Invest.*, 23:469–80.

*Acute Diarrhea: Its Nutritional Consequences
in Children*, edited by J. A. Bellanti.
Nestlé, Vevey/Raven Press, New York © 1983.

NUTRITIONAL BENEFITS RELATED TO ORAL THERAPY

Comments

M. Santosham

Johns Hopkins Project, Box 1240, Whiteriver, Arizona 85941

As discussed by Dr. Nalin (*this volume*) many questions remain unanswered in the area of nutrition related to oral therapy. The magnitude of the problem related to diarrheal disease mortality and morbidity has been pointed out by a number of authors in this volume. An example of the diarrheal disease morbidity is shown in Table 1. Approximately one-third to one-half of the children in a village in India (8) had diarrhea each month, lasting for 13 to 25% of the days in the month. Studies from Gambia (14), Mexico (3), Guatemala (10), and Bangladesh have shown a negative correlation between growth and diarrhea. Martorell et al. (9) in a longitudinal study in Guatemala estimated that the average dietary intake in infants is reduced by 160 kcal/day during a diarrheal illness in children aged 15 to 60 months (which represents about 18%–19% reduction in intake). It is clear that repeated bouts of such illness will leave a child with marginal nutritional status at a distinct nutritional disadvantage.

It is also known that the incidence of diarrheal illness tends to be higher (6) in undernourished infants compared with well nourished children in the same population (Table 2). These infants not only have a higher incidence of disease, but the disease also tends to be more severe. For example, it has been shown that in patients with cholera (12), the duration of diarrhea tends to be

TABLE 1. *Diarrheal disease incidence and duration in Punjab, India[a]*

Time period	No. episodes/ 100 children/month	Mean duration (days)
Jan–May 1971	48.0	7.4
June–Dec 1971	34.1	5.0
Jan–May 1972	47.3	5.8
June–Dec 1972	39.3	4.9
Jan–May 1973	56.3	4.0

[a] From ref. 8.

TABLE 2. *Incidence of diarrhea related to nutrition[a]*

Nutritional status	No. children observed	Weeks of observation	No. with diarrhea[b]	No. of episodes	Episodes/ 100 child/week[b]
Normal	652	7.248	187 (29%)	238	3.3
Undernourished	273	3.721	163 (40%)	286	7.7

[a] Age 0 to 23 months.
[b] $P < 0.001$.
From ref. 6.

longer (Table 3). A recent study (15) from Nigeria has also demonstrated that stunted (height/age < 75%) and underweight (weight/age < 75%) patients with noncholera diarrhea had a longer duration of diarrhea (Tables 4, 5), but had a similar incidence as normal infants. However, patients with wasting (weight/ height < 80%) had both a higher attack rate and a longer duration of diarrhea (Table 6).

The nutritional loss during diarrhea may be due to anorexia, vomiting, food withholding (which may be due to cultural habits or to a physician's instructions), altered absorption of nutrients, catabolic losses and functional wastage, i.e., diversion of nutritional resources for repair of tissues.

Dr. Nalin (*this volume*) has already reviewed the possible nutritional benefits that may be derived from oral rehydration therapy (ORT). Some of the immediate benefits of ORT have been well documented. It has been shown by several studies that rapid hydration can be achieved by using ORT alone in spite of patients presenting with history of vomiting and anorexia. Recent studies (7,11) have also demonstrated that the number of patients requiring hospitalization due to diarrheal illness can be dramatically reduced by the use of ORT. The cost saved by reducing hospitalization potentially can be diverted for nutrition programs within the community.

However, many factors remain unanswered regarding the role of introducing different types of feeding during and after the rehydration period. Balance studies in the late 1940s suggested that even though the volume and frequency of stools were greater when the child was fed, the net retention of nutrients

TABLE 3. *Severity of diarrhea and nutritional status with cholera in children*

Nutritional status	Diarrhea duration (No. of 8-hr periods)	Stool volume (Liter/kg/8 hr)
Better	7.4 ± 4.6	0.043 ± 0.032
Poorer	11.6 ± 4.4	0.063 ± 0.032

$P < 0.05$.
From ref. 12.

TABLE 4. *Attack rate and % time with diarrhea*

Ht/age	No. of children	Time with diarrhea[a]	Attack rate/child
>90%	245	7.9%	1.37
<90%	98	10.8%	1.45

[a] $P < 0.01$.
From ref. 15.

by the body also was greater (2). Pediatricians in the developed countries have suggested that a child's inability to digest lactose during a diarrheal episode may be aggravated by continued feeding of formulas containing cow's milk. However, in developing countries, the alternative of no feeding may be more damaging. There is very little information available on the relative merits of different forms of feeding during diarrheal illness. The use of lactose or non-lactose formulas, the role of continued breast-feeding, and the use of other locally available foods in different countries should be evaluated. As mentioned by Dr. Nalin, further studies also need to be conducted on the use of oral rehydration solutions (ORS) that contain substrates other than glucose to enhance the nutritional rehabilitation of patients during the acute rehydration period. These alternate solutions should also be evaluated for use in the small proportion of patients in whom the standard glucose-electrolyte solutions cannot be used due to severe malabsorption of glucose.

Dr. Nalin (*this volume*) has suggested that among the variations in the ORS composition, the most likely candidate for significant long-term nutritional benefit is prompt replacement of the potassium deficit. However, this concept remains speculative and merits further study. The optimal nutritional outcome will probably depend on a combination of factors such as the use of appropriate ORS solutions and provision of appropriate nutrients during the recovery phase of diarrhea. Finally, can any direct nutritional benefits be expected by introducing the ORS available, at present, early in the diarrheal illness? Studies from Egypt (5), Iran (1), Turkey (4), and the Philippines (13) have shown that children from communities where ORS is introduced during the early phase of diarrheal illness gained more weight when examined 1 month and 6 months

TABLE 5. *Attack rate and % time with diarrhea*

Wt/age	No. of children	Time with diarrhea[a]	Attack rate/child
>75%	220	8.5	1.25
<75%	123	11.3	1.52

[a] $P < 0.01$.
From ref. 15.

TABLE 6. *Attack rate and % time with diarrhea*

Wt/ht	No. of children	Time with diarrhea[a]	Attack rate/child[b]
>80%	302	7.6%	1.29
<80%	41	13.6%	1.90

[a] $P < 0.001$.
[b] $P < 0.02$.
From ref. 15.

later. Most of these studies were conducted in areas where the prevalence of undernutrition is high. We recently conducted a study among well nourished ambulatory children (height/weight > 3rd percentile according to National Center for Health Statistics standards) with minimal dehydration due to acute diarrhea presenting to an outpatient clinic in Panama. Patients were given either the WHO solution or one similar to the WHO solution but containing 50 mmol/liter of sodium. Children in both oral therapy groups were instructed to take the ORS *ad libitum* until diarrhea stopped and to continue their regular diet. Control patients were instructed to take a clear liquid diet consisting of the commonly available aerated beverages, bananas, cereals, and applesauce, which was the standard treatment at this clinic. Patients were seen every 24 hr until diarrhea stopped, or 2 weeks after the initial visit. The duration of diarrhea was similar in all three groups. However, we found that patients in both ORS groups gained significantly more weight compared with the control group at the time of the 2nd-week visit (Table 7). The increased weight gain seen in the ORS groups may have been due to inappropriate food-withholding in the control group, and not necessarily directly related to the use of oral rehydration. An alternate explanation is that appetite may have been restored earlier in the oral therapy groups in response to early correction of electrolyte and acid base disturbances. Additional studies are required to evaluate the long-term nutritional advantages of introducing different forms of feeding during diarrheal episodes.

TABLE 7. *Mean % weight gain after treatment in Panamanian ambulatory children with diarrhea*

No. of days after treatment	Group A[a]	Group B[b]	Group C (control)[c]
1	2.1	2.8	1.4
14[d]	5.8	6.1	3.8

[a] ORS with 90 mmol/liter Na; $n = 29$.
[b] ORS with 50 mmol/liter Na; $n = 31$.
[c] Group C (control): $n = 33$.
[d] Differences between groups A and C and groups B and C significant at $P < 0.05$.

In conclusion, although ORT has played a major role in reducing diarrheal disease mortality around the world, many questions remain unanswered about its effects on the nutritional status of children.

REFERENCES

1. Barlgar, M. A., Ourshano, S., and Amin, J. N. (1980): The evaluation of the effectiveness of oral rehydration in acute diarrhoea of children under three years of age in west Azerbaijan, Iran. *J. Trop. Pediatr.*, 26:217.
2. Chung, A. N. (1948): The effect of early oral feeding versus early starvation on the course of infantile diarrhea. *J. Pediatr.*, 33:14.
3. Condon-Paloni, D., Cravioto, J., Johnston, F. E., Delicardie, E. R., and Scholl, T. O. (1977): Morbidity and growth of infants and young children in a rural Mexican village. *Am. J. Public Health,* 67:651–656.
4. Egemen, A., and Bertan, M. (1980): A study of oral rehydration therapy by midwives in a rural area near Ankara. *Bull. WHO*, 58(2):333.
5. El-Sherbini, A. F., Fahmy, Si, Eid, E. E., Goda, M. Y., El-tantawy, A. S., and El-Sayyed, L. (1980): The use of oral rehydration in infantile diarrhea. *J. Egypt. Public Health Assoc.*, 53(Suppl. 5–6):82.
6. Ghal, O. P., and Jaiswal, V. N. (1970): Relationship of under-nutrition diarrhoea in infants and children. *Indian J. Med. Res.*, 58:789.
7. Hirschhorn, N. (1980): The treatment of acute diarrhea in children on historical and physiological perspective. *Am. J. Clin. Nutr.*, 33:637.
8. Kielmann, A., and McCord, C. (1977): Home treatment of childhood Diarrhea in Punjab villages. *Environ. Child Health*, 23:197.
9. Martorell, R., Yarbrouch, C., Yarbrough, S., and Klein, R. E. (1980): The impact of ordinary illness on the dietary intakes of malnourished children. *Am. J. Clin. Nutr.*, 33:345–350.
10. Mata, L. J., Kromal, R. A., Urrutia, J. J., and Garcia, B. (1977): Effect of infection on food intake and the nutritional state: perspectives as viewed from the village. *Am. J. Clin. Nutr.*, 30:1215–1227.
11. Oral rehydration therapy (ORT) for childhood diarrhea (1980): *Popul. Rep.*, Series L, No. 2, November-December.
12. Palmer, D. L., Koster, F. T., Alam, A. K. M. J., and Islam, M. R. (1976): Nutritional status a determinant of severity of diarrhoea in patients with cholera. *J. Infect. Dis.*, 134:8–14.
13. Report of a field trial by an international study group (1977): A positive effect on the nutrition of Philippine children of an oral glucose-electrolyte solution given at home for the treatment of diarrhoea. *Bull. WHO*, 55:87.
14. Rowland, M. G. M., Cole, T. J., and Whitehead, R. G. (1977): A quantitative study into the role of infection in determining nutritional status in Gambian village children. *Br. J. Nutr.*, 37:441–450.
15. Tomkins, A. (1981): Nutritional status and severity of diarrhoea among pre-school children in rural Nigeria. *Lancet*, 1:860–862.

Acute Diarrhea: Its Nutritional Consequences in Children, edited by J. A. Bellanti.
Nestlé, Vevey/Raven Press, New York © 1983.

NUTRITIONAL BENEFITS RELATED TO ORAL THERAPY

Discussion

Dr. Klish: It's always been my bias, as well as other people's, that the oral rehydration solutions that are on the market now need not be as nutritionally deficient as they are. The presence of glucose in these solutions is largely based on studies done in the late 1960s that showed that glucose enhances the absorption of sodium through the coupling effect in the gut mucosa. More recently, it has also been shown that the same coupling exists with amino acids.

Because of this, we have recently completed a study where we fortified oral rehydration solutions with whole protein to see what the effects on the absorption of these solutions are in perfusion models in human volunteers. We took a conventional 35 mmol sodium solution, added 1% whole whey protein to this solution, and compared the results. There was a significant enhancement of the absorption of both water and sodium as well as potassium, by as much as 50 to 60% by the addition of whey protein to the rehydration solution. Based on this, we have started some initial studies on a rehydration solution that contains protein as well as glucose and has a caloric concentration of about 0.5 calories/g. The first patients who took the solution tolerated it extremely well, and our impression was that they not only seemed to resolve as fast as on the conventional oral rehydration solution, but they may have resolved the diarrhea even faster.

Dr. Black: If we accept that there are nutritionally beneficial effects of at least most of the oral therapy intervention programs, I think we need to analyze the methodology of those programs to learn as much as we can about the effects. Two facts appear important: One is a rapid return of appetite, perhaps as a consequence of rehydration and potassium replacement; the other is that specific interventions related to education and feeding practices do take place. If we look back at the early studies in the Philippines, Turkey, and Egypt, they not only used the oral rehydration solution, but also placed heavy emphasis on early feeding and they gave very specific instructions about what should be fed.

We need oral rehydration and we need feeding; and we do not need further studies to tell us that. The important question is related to the methodology of feeding. What is optimal feeding during and after diarrhea?

Dr. Mata: I would like to ask a rather simple question and challenge a point that Dr. Santosham made in his comments.

My query relates to the statement that potassium deficits due to acute, watery diarrhea are interesting, but that their relationship to long-term nutritional damage remains speculative. This destroys the belief that most pediatricians have had that the use of potassium was one of the greatest triumphs in changing acute diarrhea from a lethal disease into one that could be managed.

Dr. Santosham: I certainly recognize that potassium is an important factor.

199

*Acute Diarrhea: Its Nutritional Consequences
in Children,* edited by J. A. Bellanti.
Nestlé, Vevey/Raven Press, New York © 1983.

PREVENTION OF ACUTE DIARRHEA IN CHILDREN

An Overview

Robert Edelman

*Clinical and Epidemiological Studies Branch, Microbiology and Infectious Diseases
Program, National Institute of Allergy and Infectious Diseases, National Institutes of
Health, Bethesda, Maryland 20205*

ENTERIC INFECTIONS

The World Health Organization published data in 1977 (41) showing that diarrhea still ranks among the leading causes of death and illness in developing countries; mortality rates in some regions continue to be as high as those of the industrial nations 80 years ago, when 4,000 per 100,000 infants died with diarrhea. From 30 to 50% of all deaths in preschool children in developing countries are associated with weaning diarrhea. In terms of morbidity, attack rates of 1.5 to 7.5 episodes of diarrhea per child per year are reported from several developing countries where reliable data are available (30). Chen estimated that from 3 to 16% of Bangladeshi children suffer from diarrhea at any given time if the average episode lasts 8 days (3). This represents an enormous burden of morbidity by any criteria, and helps to explain why diarrhea is the most important cause of nutrient wastage, restriction of calorie consumption, malnutrition, and growth retardation.

In 1979 in the United States, G. T. Curlin and J. Smith analyzed 1976 data from the National Center for Health Statistics (*unpublished data*). Diarrheal diseases accounted for 1 in 25 acute illnesses, 1 in 38 reported days of restricted activity, 1 in 63 visits to an office-based physician, and 1 in 83 (1.2%) of 38 million hospital discharges. Most of this illness is probably infectious, but, unfortunately, accurate data on etiology are not available. Traveler's diarrhea occurs in one-half of the 8 million American travelers who go overseas each year. Outbreaks of diarrhea in the 12 million children who attend day-care centers and nurseries are a growing problem. In this chapter, I have reviewed current and promising research on the prevention of the principal bacterial and viral enteropathogens responsible for this enormous burden of illness and death.

Escherichia coli

Enterotoxigenic *E. coli* (ETEC) are now known to be one of the most common causes of weanling diarrhea in the developing world, a common cause of the cholera syndrome in older children and adults living in cholera-endemic areas, and the most common identifiable cause of traveler's diarrhea (31). Fortunately, ETEC are uncommon in the United States, comprising less than 2% of the identifiable causes of diarrhea in most surveys. Currently, the identification of other *E. coli* that cause diarrhea, such as enteropathogenic *E. coli* (EPEC) and invasive *E. coli*, can be done only in reference or research laboratories. Studies of EPEC virulence have mostly been done in nursery outbreaks; whether EPEC strains are causative of sporadic cases and outbreaks of diarrhea in older children and adults is the subject of ongoing research.

Doxycycline, trimethoprim/sulfamethoxazole, or sulphadiazine/streptomycin/sulphadimidine/sulphathiazole ("streptotriad") prophylaxis has protected against ETEC-associated traveler's diarrhea in Africa and in Mexico, but practical and theoretical objections have been raised to these antibiotics as universal prophylactic agents. Effective therapy of acute diarrhea caused by ETEC has now been shown for doxycycline, trimethoprim/sulfamethoxazole, and bicozamycin, a new antibiotic that is poorly absorbed from the gastrointestinal tract.

One of the objectives of the enteric diseases programs of the National Institute of Allergy and Infectious Diseases (NIAID) and the United States Army is to develop a vaccine or vaccines against ETEC and traveler's diarrhea. Effective immunoprophylaxis will have to overcome the extreme heterogeneity of virulent ETEC strains. For example, ETEC pathogens fall into many cell wall lipopolysaccharide, capsular, and flagellar serotypes, and two or three enterotoxin phenotypes. The heat-stable enterotoxin (ST) is the toxin most commonly produced by virulent strains, but ST is not antigenic and so not amenable to vaccination (31). Moreover, although the heat-labile toxin (LT) is antigenic, volunteer studies suggest that antitoxin immunity is not the principal protective mechanism in man (24). We now know that ETEC strains must possess accessory virulence properties, in addition to enterotoxin, to cause diarrhea in man.

Veterinary work has established that most ETEC strains for young animals possess adherence or colonization factors (pili or fimbriae) that enable them to attach to mucosa of the small intestine, thereby overcoming the peristaltic defense mechanism as well as allowing release of toxin closer to susceptible epithelial cells (20). If the pili associated with human ETEC strains could be identified, purified, and shown to be immunogenic, immunoprophylaxis of ETEC disease in man should be feasible. So far, two distinct pilus antigens, CFA I and CFA II, have been identified in about 25% of human ETEC strains (20). Volunteer studies at the University of Texas at Houston with CFA I-bearing ETEC have shown that CFA I is required for multiplication of these bacteria in the intestine, for diarrhea, and for antibody response (32). Purified CFA I and CFA II pili are being prepared now as candidate vaccines for volunteer trials. Approximately 75% of ETEC strains isolated from patients carry no identified pili. If identified, epidemiological research will be required to map pili geographically so that vaccine targeted to the country traveled can be administered. Only then will we have a clear insight as to the feasibility of pili vaccines.

Our ability to diagnose ETEC-mediated disease is still relatively insensitive, and the procedures laborious. The recent publication by Moseley et al. of a rapid and specific deoxyribonucleic acid (DNA) probe technique to detect presence of the plasmid gene controlling toxin synthesis in coprobacteria promises to be an important advance (26).

Cholera

Until recently, most American clinicians regarded cholera as an exotic tropical infection of little practical importance. The reappearance of an endemic focus of cholera along the Gulf of Mexico requires that physicians familiarize themselves with the disease and its causative agent. Since 1973, isolated cases and small outbreaks of cholera have occurred in Florida, Texas, and Louisiana, and *Vibrio cholerae* El Tor Inaba was isolated from patients, from sewage and estuarine waters, and from crabs and shrimp (1).

Kaper et al. (17) have utilized molecular genetic techniques to compare *V. cholerae* isolates. The cloned gene that codes for the heat-labile toxin of *E. coli* was used as a diagnostic probe to detect the closely related cholera toxin genes isolated from American El Tor strains of *V. cholerae*. A unique, American El Tor strain, genetically distinct from El Tor and classic strains of *V. cholerae* endemic in the Eastern Hemisphere, was found to extend for hundreds of miles along the marshes of the Gulf Coast (16). We now believe that improperly cooked, contaminated, chitinous seafood serves as the vehicle by which humans contract cholera. The severity of clinical cholera depends on the number of vibrios ingested, the virulence of the organism, gastric acidity, intestinal immunity, and the blood group of exposed individuals. Severe cholera occurs more frequently in hypochlorhydric persons of blood group O. Stool specimens from persons with diarrhea following recent ingestion of crabs or shrimp should be cultured for *V. cholerae* on thiosulfate-citrate-bile-salts-sucrose agar. Cases can also be diagnosed retrospectively by serological methods. Interestingly, *V. cholerae* has also been isolated from the Chesapeake Bay, but these strains lack the enterotoxin gene and are nonpathogenic. Also, nonvirulent environmental strains do not adhere to intestinal mucosa.

The search continues for a cholera vaccine that is both safe and protective for a long duration. Starting in 1885 scientists have produced a succession of immunizing agents in a frustrating quest to produce a satisfactory vaccine against cholera. Parenteral, killed whole-cell vaccines, until recently the most intensively evaluated, were found to give variable protection of only 3 to 6 months' duration (15). More recent experiments in animals and in volunteers strongly suggest that oral immunization, rather than parenteral immunization, is the route most likely to stimulate protective intestinal immune response of the secretory IgA type (23,34). The shortcomings of parenteral immunization are that the antigen reaches intestinal lymphoid tissue inefficiently, and it stimulates suppressive mechanisms that interfere with subsequent attempts to prime or boost the immune response orally (28). Studies in Bangladesh show that parenteral immunization can boost a previously primed, local enteric response but less effectively than an oral booster (35).

Experimental cholera challenge studies done by Levine and co-workers at the Center for Vaccine Development, University of Maryland, have demonstrated that an initial clinical cholera infection of volunteers provides solid clinical and bacteriologic protection against re-challenge for at least 3 years (21). By contrast, purified, oral cholera toxoid fails to provide protection against experimental challenge with *V. cholerae* (23). Additional data in volunteers imply that antibacterial rather than antitoxin immune mechanisms predominate and limit proliferation of vibrios before they produce enterotoxin (23). These observations provide direct evidence that immunologic control of cholera may be possible if we could develop oral vaccines that mimic natural infections. The oral vaccines currently under consideration are of two classes, attenuated strains and inactivated *V. cholerae* strains combined with altered, nonreactogenic toxin, or purified toxin subunits.

An ideal, oral, attenuated cholera vaccine should be nonreactogenic, genetically stable, proliferative, and adhesive in the proximal small bowel, inductive of local antibody that prevents colonization and toxin activity, and it should stimulate long-term protection after one or two doses. No naturally occurring or laboratory-derived *V. cholerae* strain yet identified fulfills all of these criteria. However, Texas Star-SR, an attenuated mutant of a *V. cholerae* El Tor Ogawa strain prepared by Honda and Finkelstein, exhibits many qualities of an oral vaccine and has served as a prototype vaccine in volunteers (22). Texas Star-SR was obtained by nitrosoquanidine mutagenesis, and a stable clone was identified that produced ample amounts of the antigenic, intestinal binding portion of the toxin (B subunit), but only very small quantities of the toxic portion of the molecule (A subunit) (14). The strain colonized the small bowel, caused transient, low grade diarrhea in only a few volunteers, induced antitoxin or vibriocidal antibody responses in 85% of volunteers, and significantly protected volunteers against later challenge with virulent *V. cholerae* El Tor Ogawa and Inaba (22). These promising results will encourage additional effort to develop a safe and effective live, attenuated bacterial vaccine for cholera. In fact, genetic engineering and DNA recombinant techniques are being utilized now to produce better vaccine candidate strains (25).

J. Holmgren et al. (13) have produced an inactivated, oral vaccine consisting of whole vibrios and highly purified B subunits of the toxin molecule. Preliminary results in volunteers show the vaccine to be safe and antigenic (J. Holmgren, *personal communication*). In animals, the antibody produced against the lipopolysaccharide component of the whole vibrio synergizes with antitoxin to provide excellent protection (34). The combination of both antibodies is far more efficacious than the sum of the protective effect of either antibody alone. In addition, Pierce in collaboration with Germanier have fed dogs procholeragenoid, a stable high-molecular-weight aggregate of cholera toxin formed during heating of the cholera toxin (5). Procholeragenoid appears to retain full immunogenicity even though enterotoxigenicity of the molecule has been reduced by 99%. This product is safe and protects dogs against experimental cholera (29). Volunteer trials of the procholeragenoid combined with inactivated whole vibrios are being planned. The results of these vaccine studies will tell us a great deal about the virulent antigens of *V. cholerae* and the human intestinal immune response. Heretofore, most attention has been directed toward lipopolysaccharide and toxin antigens in considering immunity to *V. cholerae*. Research is underway to identify other antigens of *V. cholerae*, such as lectins, flagellar sheath material, and outer membrane proteins, that may be important in protection. The recent development by Spira et al. of a rabbit model that mimics human enterotoxigenic bacterial infections, and the rapid deployment of DNA recombinant techniques, should greatly facilitate vaccine development and testing (33).

Typhoid Fever and Other Bacterial Enteric Infections

Typhoid fever remains a serious public health problem in many regions of the world. The available parenteral typhoid vaccines are neither entirely safe nor fully protective (40). Thus, the recent development and successful field tests of a live, oral typhoid vaccine by Germanier represents an exciting advance (8). This vaccine consists of a mutagenized strain of *Salmonella typhi* (Ty21a) that is incapable of utilizing galactose after this sugar enters the bacterium. The galactose accumulates in the cell and eventually kills it in 3 to 5 days. But during that time the strain successfully proliferates and immunizes the bowel. The vaccine was tested in animals and in volunteers at the University of Maryland before it was given to 16,000 Egyptian school children (40). The strain, administered in three doses as a live, lyophilized oral vaccine, safely protected 95% of the school children against typhoid fever over a 3-year followup period (39). Black found that the vaccine apparently immunizes equally well after one dose in an enteric-coated capsule, and a field trial in Chile of this more practical dose schedule is planned (R. E. Black, *personal communication*).

Shigella sonnei and *S. flexneri* together cause 80% of the cases of bacillary dysentery worldwide and they remain a problem on Indian reservations and institutional populations in the United States. *Shigella* can infect man and cause dysentery in very small doses of 10^1 to 10^2 organisms; other bacterial pathogens require an inoculum of 1,000 to 10,000 times that dose. Until now, oral, killed and attenuated vaccine candidates have lacked necessary safety, stability, or efficacy (7). Using genetic engineering, Formal and co-workers have inserted plasmid genes coding for the protective antigen on *S. sonnei* into the *S. typhi* Ty21a strain (6). The resulting mutant organism was found to be stable and protect mice against challenge with either *S. typhi* or *S. sonnei*. These exciting data suggest that the Ty21a oral vaccine strain may be a useful carrier of antigens to protect against other enteric pathogens. Based on this strategy, an "all-purpose" oral, attenuated dysentery vaccine is under development at the Walter Reed Army Institute of Research.

A final enteric pathogen deserves recognition and comment. *Campylobacter fetus* subsp. *jejuni* often causes an enteritis more frequently than do *Salmonella* and *Shigella* in the United States and overseas; it may account for 5 to 11% of all cases of diarrhea (2). Most *Campylobacter* isolates are obtained in the summer and fall from older children and young adults. A selective culture medium, initially developed in Belgium, allows prompt isolation of the organism. Erythromycin or doxycycline therapy, if started early enough, would seem effective for chronic or severe cases. But the large number of serotypes discovered so far, and the absence of information about clinical immunity, mode of transmission, contagiousness, and pathogenic mechanisms, makes attempts to develop immunoprophylaxis premature.

Norwalk Virus

Prior to 1972, studies of infants and young children hospitalized with sporadic or epidemic diarrhea and vomiting failed to uncover a causative agent. Then Dolin and Kapikian at the NIAID prepared a filtrate of a rectal swab from a patient with acute gastroenteritis in Norwalk, Ohio, and examined this infectious stool filtrate by immune electron microscopy (IEM) using convalescent serum (19). Twenty-seven nm particles resembling parvoviruses, subsequently named Norwalk virus, were aggregated by the antiserum under the electron microscope. Kapikian was able to demonstrate serological evidence of infection by IEM, and a close temporal relationship between illness and the presence of the Norwalk virus in stools during experimental infection.

The development of a radioimmunoassay (RIA) for Norwalk virus in 1978 by Greenberg et al. was the next major advance that has enabled better elucidation of the role of Norwalk virus in viral gastroenteritis (12). RIA more readily permitted detection of virus in feces and measurement of serum antibody. It now appears that Norwalk virus causes approximately one-third of the epidemics of acute, nonbacterial gastroenteritis in the United States, and young children are not commonly involved; overseas, it is associated with endemic and epidemic gastroenteritis in all age groups (10,11). Epidemic transmission of the virus has occurred via contaminated drinking and swimming water, and contaminated oysters and lettuce. Airborne transmission may occur. The illness, characterized by diarrhea or vomiting or both signs, is usually self-limited and characteristically lasts only 24 to 48 hr. Norwalk virus may cause mild gastroenteritis in young children overseas, but there is no evidence that Norwalk virus affects young children in the United States except during epidemics. Interestingly enough, when volunteers were inoculated with Norwalk virus and then rechallenged 2 to 3½ years later, precisely the same volunteers who became ill on the first challenge became ill again (27). Those who were clinically well on the first challenge remained so on the second. The antibody response is another unusual and striking feature of Norwalk gastroenteritis. Paradoxically, and in contrast with other viral infections, the presence of serum and jejunal antibody to the virus and the ability to produce antibody constitute a risk factor for illness.

The Norwalk virus is actually the prototype and most extensively studied strain of a group of noncultivatable agents that we now call Norwalk-like viruses. Definitive classification and characterization of these viruses awaits determination of their nucleic acid content and antigenic structure; this information, in turn, awaits *in vitro* propagation to accumulate enough virus for research. Unlike rotavirus, Norwalk virus is shed in human stool in relatively small amounts. Routine diagnostic tests are urgently needed, because IEM and RIA are cumbersome and restricted to a few research laboratories. Suitable reagents are scarce and difficult to obtain, thus preventing the preparation of purified virus and serological reagents for diagnostic purposes.

Immediate prospects for a Norwalk virus vaccine appear dim for several reasons. Animal models of Norwalk virus infection and diarrhea do not exist; the virus cannot be propagated *in vitro*; and the confusing, atypical pattern of clinical immunity observed in this illness obviates any rational immunization schedule.

Rotavirus

Studies in the United States and overseas have shown the rotaviruses of the family Reoviridae to be major pathogens of infants under 2 years of age (18). Overall rotaviruses cause one-half of the cases of severe diarrhea, dehydration, and fever requiring hospitalization in this age group. In adults, rotavirus has been associated with traveler's diarrhea and outbreaks of acute gastroenteritis. The control of rotaviral infections represents an important and worldwide public health challenge. Since its discovery in 1973, there has been an explosion of knowledge about rotavirus, and unlike Norwalk virus, many of the biological, clinical, pathogenetic, and epidemiologic characteristics are reasonably well understood. Unfortunately, efforts at immunoprophylaxis have been hampered by the inability to propagate human rotaviruses serially to high titer *in vitro*. Recently, Wyatt and co-workers (42) serially propagated human type 2 rotavirus in cell culture after it had undergone 11 serial passages in gnotobiotic piglets. This virus strain has been grown in amounts sufficient for laboratory characterization. The virus was attenuated during passage and represents the first, oral rotavirus vaccine candidate. Safety and antigenicity studies of the vaccine strain, called WA, are now proceeding in adult volunteers at the University of Maryland and at the NIAID.

Except for the WA strain, most human and many mammalian rotavirus strains undergo an abortive infection in cell culture in which viral antigens are produced without release of infectious virus. In an important development, Greenberg et al. (9) converted fastidious rotaviruses into viruses capable of efficient growth in tissue culture by mixing human rotaviruses with a cultivatable bovine rotavirus in cell culture. The segmented genes of the noncultivable human rotavirus that restricts growth *in vitro* were replaced by the growth-permissive genes of the bovine rotavirus without replacing the genes that determine the antigens on the human virus. In this manner poorly growing human rotavirus can be grown and recovered in titers sufficiently high for laboratory characterization. In addition to its use for viral recovery and diagnosis, it may be possible to construct, through gene reassortment during coinfection, attenuated rotavirus vaccine candidates. The genes controlling for virulence or attenuation also can be identified and manipulated in this way.

The production of monoclonal antibodies to rotavirus proteins, now underway at the NIAID and elsewhere, will be most useful for large scale epidemiological studies using a variety of serological tests, including CF, enzyme-linked immunosorbent assay (ELISA), immunofluorescence, immune adherence hemagglutination assay, and plaque reduction neutralization. Knowledge of the distinct human rotavirus serotypes and subgroups is necessary for planning an effective vaccine strategy. However, at present, the number of human rotavirus serotypes of medical importance is uncertain.

A large proportion of children infected with the human rotavirus develop antibodies against bovine rotavirus in addition to the infecting human virus. In addition, prior exposure of calves to calf-derived rotavirus protects them against experimental challenge with human rotavirus, which would normally produce disease (43). Thus, it might be possible to immunize children similarly against human rotavirus disease utilizing the calf virus if it infects humans asymptomatically while inducing clinical immunity. Preliminary data suggest that resistance to rotavirus disease in volunteers challenged with rotavirus is most clearly associated with the level of type-specific rotavirus antibody in their serum and intestinal secretions (18). Breast-feeding also protects against rotavirus diarrhea in infants; this effect may be due to secretory IgA rotavirus antibodies and to other protective factors in milk (37). Pooled human breast milk is being fed to infants to control outbreaks of rotavirus diarrhea in hospitals. Proposals to add bovine anti-rotavirus immunoglobulin to infant formulas have been under review by the United States Food and Drug Administration.

Although a number of morphologically different viruses and virus-like particles have been pictured by electron microscopy in diarrheal stools, except for rotavirus and the Norwalk agent, the lack of epidemiological evidence has foiled attempts to link them causally with gastroenteritis. However, two newly identified viruses, calicivirus and enteral adenoviruses, are now emerging as additional agents of viral gastroenteritis.

Calicivirus

Caliciviruses have been found in the stools of infants in an orphanage in Japan, where the correlation between viral shedding and the days of illness was clearly demonstrated; namely, no virus shedders before illness, 95% virus shedders within 4 days of illness, 50% from the fifth to the ninth day, and <10% thereafter (4). The illness in these infants was milder than that seen in rotavirus infections, although vomiting and fever characterized outbreaks of apparent calicivirus diarrhea in older children in England. Antigenic comparison between strains and serological and epidemiological descriptions await the successful propagation of the virus *in vitro*.

Adenovirus

Fastidious adenoviruses that do not grow readily in conventional cell culture systems have been detected by electron microscopy in up to 5% of stools of infants and young children hospitalized with diarrhea (18). The adenovirus-associated diarrhea has usually been mild, but severe dehydration, intussusception, and death have been reported. The virus has appeared in Europe, North America, and India. Using virions purified directly from diarrheal stools, Wadell et al. (38) have characterized these noncultivable agents as members of a new subgroup of adenovirus. Using an ELISA for detection of adenovirus antigen in stool, Yolken et al. (44) have linked these fastidious viruses with a large, hospital-associated outbreak of severe respiratory infections and diarrhea. The recent propagation of these enteral adenoviruses by Takiff et al. (36) in an adenovirus type 5 transformed human embryonic kidney cell line will surely provide the reagents needed to examine enteral adenovirus epidemiology and pathogenicity more thoroughly.

CONCLUSION

Epidemiological research has been hampered by the absence of simple and rapid techniques to identify ETEC and gastrointestinal viruses other than rotavirus. With the recent advent of DNA recombinant techniques and monoclonal antibodies, it should be possible to improve diagnosis and learn more about the epidemiology of these diarrheal diseases. With the newer understanding of intestinal immunity and genetic engineering, we can soon gain insight into pathogenic mechanisms and ways to devise vaccines that will contain appropriate virulence factors necessary for broad-spectrum protection. Already, new, oral vaccines against typhoid fever, ETEC, cholera, and rotavirus disease have progressed to the stage of human testing. If logistical problems can be overcome, some of these vaccines should help alleviate the nutrient wastage, restriction of calories, and growth retardation experienced by so many pre-school children, particularly those living in developing countries.

REFERENCES

1. Blake, P. A., Allegra, D. T., Snyder, J. D., Barrett, T. J., McFarland, L., Caraway, C. T., Feeley, J. C., Craig, J. P., Lee, J. V., Puhr, N. D., and Feldman, R. A. (1980): Cholera—a possible endemic focus in the United States. *N. Engl. J. Med.*, 302:305–309.
2. Blaser, M. J., and Reller, L. B. (1981): *Campylobacter* enteritis. *N. Engl. J. Med.*, 305:1444–1452.
3. Chen, L. C. (1978): Control of diarrheal disease morbidity and mortality: Some strategic issues. In: *Proceedings of a National Academy of Sciences Workshop on Effective Interventions to Reduce Infections in Malnourished Populations*, edited by G. T. Keusch and M. Katz. *Am. J. Clin. Nutr.*, 31:2284–2291.
4. Chiba, S., Sakuma, Y., Kogasaka, R., Akihara, M., Terashima, H., Horino, K., and Nakao, T. (1980): Fecal shedding of virus in relation to the days of illness in infantile gastroenteritis due to calicivirus. *J. Infect. Dis.*, 142:247–249.
5. Finkelstein, R. A., Fujita, K., and LoSpalluto, J. J. (1971): Procholeragenoid: An aggregated intermediate in the formation of choleragenoid. *J. Immunol.*, 107:1043–1051.
6. Formal, S. B., Baron, L. S., Kopecko, D. J., Washington, O., Powell, C., and Life, C. A. (1981): Construction of a potential bivalent vaccine strain: Introduction of *Shigella sonnei* form I antigen genes into the galE *Salmonella typhi* Ty21a typhoid vaccine strain. *Infect. Immun.*, 34:746–750.
7. Formal, S. B., Maenza, R. M., Austin, S., and LaBree, E. H. (1967): Failure of parenteral vaccines to protect monkeys against experimental shigellosis. *Proc. Soc. Exp. Biol. Med.*, 125:347–349.
8. Germanier, R. (1981): W.H.O. diarrhoeal diseases control programme. Present status of immunization against typhoid fever. *World Health Organization*, WHO/CDD/BEI/81.3, pp. 1–14.
9. Greenberg, H. B., Kalica, A. R., Wyatt, R. G., Jones, R. W., Kapikian, A. Z., and Chanock, R. M. (1981): Rescue of non-cultivatable human rotavirus by gene reassortment during mixed infection with *ts* mutants of a cultivatable bovine rotavirus. *Proc. Natl. Acad. Sci. USA*, 78:420–424.
10. Greenberg, H. B., Valdesuso, J., Kapikian, A. Z., Chanock, R. M., Wyatt, R. G., Szmuness, W., Larrick, J., Kaplan, J., Gilman, R. H., and Sack, D. A. (1979): Prevalence of antibody to the Norwalk virus in various countries. *Infect. Immun.*, 26:270–273.
11. Greenberg, H. B., Valdesuso, J., Yolken, R. H., Gangarosa, E., Gary, W., Wyatt, R. G., Konno, T., Suzuki, H., Chanock, R. M., and Kapikian, A. Z. (1979): Role of Norwalk virus in outbreaks of nonbacterial gastroenteritis. *J. Infect. Dis.*, 139:564–568.
12. Greenberg, H. B., Wyatt, R. G., Valdesuso, J., Kalica, A. R., London, W. T., Chanock, R. M., and Kapikian, A. Z. (1978): Solid-phase microtiter radioimmunoassay for detection of the Norwalk strain of acute nonbacterial, epidemic gastroenteritis virus and its antibodies. *J. Med. Virol.*, 2:97–108.
13. Holmgren, J., Svennerholm, A.-M., Lonnroth, I., Fall-Persson, M., Markman, B., and Lundback, H. (1977): Development of improved cholera vaccine based on subunit toxoid. *Nature*, 269:602–604.
14. Honda, T., and Finkelstein, R. A. (1979): Selection and characteristics of a *Vibrio cholerae* mutant lacking the A [ADP-ribosylating] portion of the cholera enterotoxin. *Proc. Natl. Acad. Sci. USA*, 76:2052–2056.
15. Joo, I. (1974): Cholera vaccines. In: *Cholera*, edited by D. Barma and W. Burrows, pp. 333–355. Saunders, Philadelphia.
16. Kaper, J. B., Bradford, H. B., Roberts, N. C., and Falcow, S. (1982): Molecular epidemiology of *Vibrio cholerae* in the U.S. Gulf Coast. *J. Clin. Microbiol.*, 16:129–134.
17. Kaper, J. B., Moseley, S. L., and Falcow, S. (1981): Molecular characterization of environmental and nontoxigenic strains of *Vibrio cholerae. Infect. Immun.*, 32:661–667.
18. Kapikian, A. Z., Greenberg, H. B., Kalica, A. R., Wyatt, R. G., Kim, H. W., Brandt, C. D., Rodriguez, W. J., Flores, J., Singh, N., Parrott, R. H., and Chanock, R. M. (1981): New developments in viral gastroenteritis. In: *Acute Enteric Infections in Children. New Prospects for Treatment and Prevention*, edited by T. Holme, J. Holmgren, M. H. Merson, and R. Mollby, pp. 9–57. Elsevier/North-Holland, Amsterdam.

19. Kapikian, A. Z., Wyatt, R. G., Dolin, R., Thornhill, T. S., Kalica, A. R., Chanock, R. M. (1972): Visualization by immune electronmicroscopy of a 27-nm particle associated with acute infectious nonbacterial gastroenteritis. *J. Virol.*, 10:1075–1081.
20. Levine, M. M. (1981): Adhesion of enterotoxigenic *Escherichia coli* in humans and animals. In: *Adhesion and Microorganism Pathogenicity*, edited by K. Elliot, M. O'Connor, and J. Whelan, pp. 142–154. Ciba Foundation Symposium 80, Pitman Press, Bath, England.
21. Levine, M. M., Black, R. E., Clements, M. L., Cisneros, L., Nalin, D. R., and Young, C. R. (1981): Duration of infection-derived immunity to cholera. *J. Infect. Dis.*, 143:818–820.
22. Levine, M. M., Black, R. E., Clements, M. L., Young, C. R., Honda, T., and Finkelstein, R. A. (1983): Texas Star-SR: Attenuated *Vibrio cholerae* oral vaccine candidate. In: *Proceedings of the 17th Joint Conference on Cholera, U.S.-Japan Cooperative Medical Science Program* (in Press).
23. Levine, M. M., Nalin, D. R., Craig, J. P., Hoover, D., Bergquist, E. J., Waterman, D., Holley, H. P., Hornick, R. B., Pierce, N. P., and Libonati, J. P. (1979): Immunity of cholera in man: Relative role of antibacterial versus antitoxic immunity. *Trans. R. Soc. Trop. Med. Hyg.*, 73:3–9.
24. Levine, M. M., Nalin, D. R., Hoover, D. L., Bergquist, E. J., Hornick, R. B., Young, C. R. (1979): Immunity to enterotoxigenic *Escherichia coli*. *Infect. Immun.*, 23:729–736.
25. Mekalanos, J. J., Moseley, S. L., Murphy, J. R., and Falkow, S. (1982): Isolation of enterotoxin structural gene deletion mutations in *Vibrio cholerae* induced by two mutagenic vibriophages. *Proc. Natl. Acad. Sci. USA*, 79:151–155.
26. Moseley, S. L., Echeverria, P., Seriwatana, J., Tirapat, C., Chaicumpa, W., Sakuldaipeara, T., and Falcow, S. (1982): Identification of enterotoxigenic *Escherichia coli* by colony hybridization using three enterotoxin gene probes. *J. Infect. Dis.*, 145:863–869.
27. Parrino, T. A., Schreiber, D. S., Trier, J. S., Kapikian, A. Z., Blacklow, N. R. (1977): Clinical immunity in acute gastroenteritis caused by Norwalk agent. *N. Engl. J. Med.*, 297:86–89.
28. Pierce, N. F. (1980): Suppression of the intestinal immune response to cholera toxin by specific serum antibody. *Infect. Immun.*, 30:62–68.
29. Pierce, N. F., Cray, W. C., Jr., Sacci, J. B., Jr., and Germanier, R. (1983): Oral immunization for cholera: Mucosal antitoxic immunity is important and can probably be safely achieved. In: *Recent Progress in Cholera Research. Proceedings of the 17th Joint Conference on Cholera, U.S.-Japan Cooperative Medical Science Program*, edited by S. Kuwahara and N. F. Pierce. KTK Scientific Publishers, Tokyo.
30. Rohde, J. E. (1978): Preparing for the next round: Convalescent care after acute infection. In: *Proceedings of a National Academy of Sciences Workshop on Effective Interventions to Reduce Infections in Malnourished Populations*, edited by G. T. Keusch and M. Katz. *Am. J. Clin. Nutr.*, 31:2258–2268.
31. Sack, R. B. (1980): Enterotoxigenic *Escherichia coli*: Identification and characterization. *J. Infect. Dis.*, 142:279–286.
32. Satterwhite, T. K., Evans, D. G., Dupont, H. L., and Evans, D. J., Jr. (1978): Role of *Escherichia coli* colonisation factor antigen in acute diarrhea. *Lancet*, ii:181–184.
33. Spira, W. M., Sack, R. B., and Froehlich, J. L. (1981): Simple adult rabbit model for *Vibrio cholerae* and enterotoxigenic *Escherichia coli* diarrhea. *Infect. Immun.*, 32:739–747.
34. Svennerholm, A.-M., and Holmgren, J. (1976): Synergistic protective effect in rabbits of immunization with *Vibrio cholerae* lipopolysaccharide and toxin/toxoids. *Infect. Immun.*, 13:735–740.
35. Svennerholm, A.-M., Sack, D. A., Holmgren, J., and Bardhan, P. K. (1982): Intestinal antibody responses after immunisation with cholera B subunit. *Lancet*, i:305–308.
36. Takiff, H. E., Straus, S. E., and Garon, C. F. (1981): Propagation and *in vitro* studies of previously non-cultivable enteral adenoviruses in 293 cells. *Lancet*, ii:832–834.
37. Totterdell, B. M., Chrystie, I. L., Banatvala, J. E. (1980): Cord blood and breast milk antibodies in neonatal rotavirus infection. *Br. Med. J.*, 280:828–830.
38. Wadell, G., Hammarskjuld, M. L., Winberg, G., Varsanyi, T. M., and Sundell, G. (1980): Genetic variability of adenoviruses. *Ann. NY Acad. Sci.*, 354:16–42.
39. Wahdan, M. H., Serie, C., Cerisier, Y., Sallam, S., and Germanier, R. (1982): A controlled field trial of live *Salmonella typhi* strain Ty21a oral vaccine against typhoid: Three-year results. *J. Infect. Dis.*, 145:292–295.

40. Woodward, W. E. (1980): Volunteer studies of typhoid fever and vaccines. *Trans. R. Soc. Trop. Med. Hyg.*, 74:553–556.
41. World Health Organization (1977): New knowledge and research needs in the control of acute diarrhoeal diseases. WHO (ACMR 19/77.13), Geneva.
42. Wyatt, R. G., James, W. D., Bahl, E. H., Theil, K. W., Saif, L. J., Kalica, A. R., Greenberg, H. B., Kapikian, A. Z., and Chanock, R. M. (1980): Human rotavirus types 2: Cultivation *in vitro. Science*, 207:189–191.
43. Wyatt, R. G., Kapikian, A. Z., Greenberg, H. B., Kalica, A. R., and Chanock, R. M. (1981): Prospects for development of a vaccine against rotavirus diarrhea. In: *Acute Enteric Infections in Children. New Prospects for Treatment and Prevention*, edited by T. Holme, J. Holmgren, M. H. Merson, and R. Mollby, pp. 505–522. Elsevier/North-Holland, Amsterdam.
44. Yolken, R. H., Lawrence, F., Leister, F., Takiff, H. E., and Straus, S. E. (1982): Gastroenteritis associated with enteric type adenovirus in hospitalized infants. *J. Pediatr.*, 101:21–26.

Acute Diarrhea: Its Nutritional Consequences in Children, edited by J. A. Bellanti.
Nestlé, Vevey/Raven Press, New York © 1983.

PREVENTION OF ACUTE DIARRHEA IN CHILDREN

Comments

José O. Mora

Department of Community Medicine, Columbian School of Medicine, Bogota, Columbia

The prevention of acute diarrhea, particularly in childhood, is a world challenge (14). As happens with most socially induced health problems resulting from inequity and poverty, its root causes are difficult to overcome, and its prevention is not a straightforward and easy task. The multifactorial nature of the etiology of acute diarrhea at the community level poses a major obstacle to prevention.

It is not by coincidence that the prevention of acute diarrhea in childhood shares many conceptual and operational problems with the prevention of infant malnutrition. The two conditions, besides their common social etiology, are usually and deeply associated in a two-way cause-and-effect relationship. Under these circumstances, the assessment of their direct and immediate causative agents (viral, bacterial, or parasitic agents in diarrhea, or specific nutrient deficiencies in malnutrition), although important, does not seem to have the highest relevance for prevention, and the controversy is still valid as to the cost-effectiveness of the holistic approach versus narrowly targeted interventions (6).

The conceptual basis for the prevention of acute diarrhea stems basically from its major epidemiologic characteristics: distribution in time, place, and person, and basic mechanisms of transmission. Seasonal variations, association with unsanitary places and practices, preference for early childhood, and the fecal-oral mode of transmission are key features (13). Preventive strategies should, therefore, deal with the sanitary environment, as well as with all elements implicated in the process leading to ingestion of fecally contaminated materials by the unprotected small child (12). On these grounds, prevention of acute diarrhea may be conceptualized at the primary or at the secondary level.

PRIMARY PREVENTION

Prevention at the primary level involves all actions aimed at the interruption of the mechanism of transmission at the "source" level, throughout the process of transportation of contaminated materials to the host, and at the host level, e.g., measures to prevent contaminated materials (water, food, etc.) from being ingested by the child. Most of the preventive measures at the primary level relate to environmental sanitation at the community and household level, but others are addressed directly to the host. Basic environmental sanitation measures at the community and household level have been traditionally regarded as the only ones likely to produce enduring preventive effects.

Since contaminated water plays an important role in the transmission of enteropathogens, the provision of readily available potable water has been viewed as the major preventive measure. However, many major capital intensive water improvement schemes have been ineffective in reducing diarrheal morbidity. It seems that the quality and usage pattern of water in the home, not just the quality of water at its source, largely determine the incidence of diarrheal morbidity in individual members of the community, particularly the children. The provision of safe drinking water alone is not sufficient to prevent acute diarrheal diseases; furthermore, it is often highly expensive, compromising possible investments in other equally or more effective interventions (1,11).

The safe disposal of human feces should lead to substantial reductions in transmission of many of the diarrheal disease agents, with a corresponding reduction of morbidity (9). Effectiveness of these sanitation schemes for excreta and sewage disposal is, however, contingent on their appropriateness to the culturally determined behavioral patterns of the community, and the implementation of effective education toward optimal use of the facilities, as well as on the active community participation in their implementation.

Preventive Measures at the Host Level

Most preventive measures at the host level are likely to be implementable through appropriate education. They are not only the least expensive but also, probably, the most effective to reduce the incidence of acute diarrhea in children (3). They should have three major objectives: these are described below.

Preventing Fecal Contamination of Drinking Water and Foods at the Household and Individual Level

1. Hygienic water treatment at the house-hold level (boiling or other treatment methods) is required.
2. With prepared food, appropriate practices of food conservation, handling, and protection are necessary. Fly control may play an important role in this regard, as well as hand-washing and other personal hygienic practices.

Preventing Contaminated Materials from Being Ingested by the Child

1. Any measures to promote breast-feeding will reduce the opportunities for the child's exposure to contaminated foods. Prolonged breast-feeding ap-

pears to be the single most effective measure to prevent diarrhea in children, with a key direct role up to 6 months, and an indirect effect over the period of highest incidence throughout the second semester and into the second year of life (8). While the direct effect is mostly due to the increasingly known antiinfectious properties of breast milk, the indirect effect is due to both the reduction of the opportunities for the child's exposure to ingestion of contaminated foods and the contribution of breast-feeding to maintain a good nutritional status of the child (4).

2. Delayed introduction of supplementary foods in the child's diet is useful, both to reduce the chances of ingestion of contaminated foods and to facilitate the promotion of prolonged breast-feeding. There seems to be enough evidence to sustain that, under appropriate breast feeding patterns, introduction of supplementary foods before the fourth month is not only unnecessary, but may also carry a high risk of exposure to contamination, particularly in unsanitary environments.

3. Provision of safe weaning foods and practices is required. Since contaminated weaning foods have been identified as major vehicles for the transmission of fecal pathogens during early infancy, appropriated technologies for weaning foods have been advocated as an important preventive measure (2). These may include the preparation of dry ingredients, better cooking and feeding practices, and changes in consumption patterns, such as reducing the standing time of already cooked weaning foods and avoiding the use of bottle-feeding, as much as possible, in favor of spoon-feeding.

Increasing the Child's Resistance to the Infectious Agents of Acute Diarrhea

1. Prolonged breast-feeding will increase the immunity.

2. To prevent the reduction of immunity, it is necessary to improve the nutritional status, from pregnancy on throughout the prenatal and postnatal period of high risk.

3. A basic measure to meet the objective is to improve active immunity, particularly intestinal secretory antibody immunity, through immunoprophylaxis. Prospects for vaccine development against the most common bacterial and viral agents of acute diarrhea are promising, particularly oral vaccines against salmonellae, shigellas, and rotaviruses (15). The development of a rotavirus vaccine is considered by WHO to be of high priority in designing a strategy for immunoprophylaxis against acute diarrhea in infancy and early childhood, which has been shown to be associated with such viral agents in up to 80% of the cases (5,10). The practical relevance of the vaccines eventually developed will depend, to a great extent, on the relative contribution of the known enteropathogens to the etiology of acute diarrhea in a given setting. Studies in this regard will be highly relevant to the extensive use and expected cost-effectiveness of immunizations for the prevention of acute diarrhea.

SECONDARY PREVENTION

The outcome of diarrheal disease may be greatly influenced by management of the acute case, providing an opportunity to prevent some of the sequelae. These include appropriate treatment and measures to prevent and/or correct dehydration through early oral rehydration therapy (7), as well as those to avoid serious nutritional impairment, such as uninterrupted breast-feeding, shortened period of dietary restrictions, measures to control anorexia (e.g., oral rehydration therapy), and early and appropriate refeeding. It is recognized that therapeutic actions are, in some sense, also essential components of prevention.

REFERENCES

1. Briscoe, J. (1978): The role of water supply in improving health in poor countries (with special reference to Bangladesh). *Am. J. Clin. Nutr.*, 31:2100–2113.
2. Brown, R. E. (1978): Weaning foods in developing countries. *Am. J. Clin. Nutr.*, 31:2066–2072.
3. Chen, L. C. (1978): Control of diarrheal disease morbidity and mortality: some strategic issues. *Am. J. Clin. Nutr.*, 31:2284–2291.
4. Cunningham, A. S. (1979): Morbidity in breast-fed and artificially fed infants II. *J. Pediatr.*, 95:685–689.
5. Konno, T., Suzuki, H., and Imar, A. A. (1978): A long term study of rotavirus infections in Japanese children with acute gastroenteritis. *J. Infect. Dis.*, 138:569–576.
6. Latham, M. C. (1978): Strategies to control infections in malnourished populations—holistic approach or narrowly targeted interventions. *Am. J. Clin. Nutr.*, 31:2292–2300.
7. Mahalanabis, D., Merson, M. H., and Barua, D. (1981): Oral rehydration therapy—recent advances. *World Health Forum*, 2(2):245–249.
8. Mata, L. J. (1978): Breast-feeding: main promoter of infant health. *Am. J. Clin. Nutr.*, 31:2058–2065.
9. McCabe, L. J., and Haines, T. W. (1957): Diarrhoeal disease control by improved human excreta disposal. *Public Health Rep.*, 72:921–928.
10. Metselaar, D., Sack, D. A., and Kapikian, A. Z. (1978): Agents affecting health of mother and child in a rural area of Kenya. *Trop. Geogr. Med.*, 30(4):531–535.
11. Schneider, R. E., Shiffman, M., and Faigenblum, J. (1978): The potential effect of water on gastrointestinal infections prevalent in developing countries. *Am. J. Clin. Nutr.*, 31:2089–2099.
12. United Nations University (1982): Prevention and control of diarrhoeal diseases. *Food Nutr. Bull.*, 4(1):17–19.
13. Van Zijl, W. J. (1966): Studies on diarrheal diseases in seven countries by the WHO Diarrheal Diseases Advisory Team. *Bull. WHO*, 35:249–261.
14. World Health Organization (1978): *Development of a Programme for Diarrhoeal Disease Control.* WHO/DDC/78.1, Geneva.
15. World Health Organization (1980): *Programme for Control of Diarrhoeal Diseases.* Scientific Working Group Reports, 1978–1980. WHO/CDD/80.1, Geneva.

Acute Diarrhea: Its Nutritional Consequences in Children, edited by J. A. Bellanti.
Nestlé, Vevey/Raven Press, New York © 1983.

PREVENTION OF ACUTE DIARRHEA IN CHILDREN

Discussion

Dr. Robbins: I would like to make some unrelated comments about the problem of vaccines designed to prevent diarrheal disease. The first comment comes from our experience with the use of pneumococcal vaccine to treat pneumonia. We are entering an age where the diseases that we are going to prevent are caused by a variety of agents. We no longer have vaccines with high degrees of specificity, such as against diphtheria or tetanus. We are now attempting to treat diarrhea, which has many etiologies.

In the case of the pneumococcal vaccine designed to prevent pneumonia, pneumococci comprise only a fraction of the etiologic agents that can cause pneumonia, so that if a prevention program for diarrheal diseases is going to be attempted, the overall problem of diarrhea also has to be considered when the individual etiologic agents are being studied. This will mean complex vaccines, and it will also mean that laboratories—the national control laboratories and the investigative laboratories that are studying the effects of the individual vaccine and the entire problem of diarrhea—will have to be equipped with the diagnostic and serologic facilities for studying many diseases. This will pose new problems for the study of vaccines that have not been anticipated previously.

Polio virus is an interesting example of an enteric disease and how the development of vaccines in this field has altered over the years. Polio is a virus that colonizes the intestinal tract and, in a small proportion of people, it escapes into the circulation and infects the anterior horn cells. The disease is myelitis, but the initial infection is in the enteric tract. The first vaccines were preparations of polio virus that were inactivated, so that they would no longer be infective; these were effective vaccines. They were not very immunogenic because of the difficulty of preparing large amounts of polio virus. The second development in the field, of course, was the development of the oral, attenuated strains. These were extraordinarily effective and a remarkable advance in medicine and science, but they do pose three problems. The first is that they are living viruses and are susceptible to high temperatures; therefore they must be protected in a controlled environment. The second is that they cannot be given to many children too early, because if the children are nursing, breast milk will inhibit the replication of the virus. And the third, and not so well understood, is the problem of interference when the virus is given to some children who have active infections. It has been proposed that the inability to colonize and immunize some children might be due to interferon levels, or other antiviral reactants that are going under active inflammation.

In Holland about 15 years ago, they set out to develop inactivated polio virus by new technologies. They have achieved a stunning success, so that their new vaccine contains many more antigens than the previous vaccines. One injection is sufficient to give enough protective antibodies, so that you could predict that the child will be protected for life, and the injection can be given in infants and children as young as 2 to 3 months of age. There are many advantages to this material. It's more heat-resistant, it can immunize young infants, and it seems to be independent of the inflammatory stage of the gastrointestinal tract.

I mention this because it does give a different view of immunization and leads also into another problem—immunization problems per se. We are all aware how difficult it is to have an effective immunization program where at least 90 to 95% of the children participate. Therefore, the prospect of introducing additional vaccines that cannot be given simultaneously with our current ones raises problems of cost, delivery, care, etc. It would be ideal if the diarrheal vaccines could be made so that they could be given with our current vaccine programs and not add to the cost and to the other problems entailed in the delivery of additional vaccines.

Subject Index